Life with Alzheimer's

And the Wonderful
"Moments in Time"

By Trisha Waskey

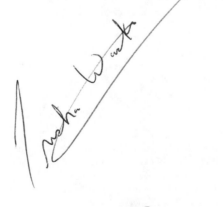

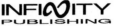

INFINITY
PUBLISHING

Copyright © 2009 by Trisha Waskey

Interior Artwork: Joanne Newman

ISBN 0-7414-5855-1

Library of Congress Control Number: 2009907065

Printed in the United States of America

Published May 2010

∞

INFINITY PUBLISHING
1094 New DeHaven Street, Suite 100
West Conshohocken, PA 19428-2713
Toll-free (877) BUY BOOK
Local Phone (610) 941-9999
Fax (610) 941-9959
Info@buybooksontheweb.com
www.buybooksontheweb.com

Contents

Introduction

Throughout our lives, from the moment we are conceived, we create memories. As we grow older, the number of memories we have increases. We surround ourselves with family and friends, with work and play, and we are continuously adding to our file of memories... the *treasures* belonging only to us, which make us who we are.

There is joy in reminiscing, laughter from stories told and retold, comfort in the pictures of the ones we love and pain in the memories we'd like to forget. But all these memories, these *treasures,* are tucked away in our *treasure box* (our brain). They are pulled out, just as a toy would be out of a toy chest, and we find comfort in the familiarity of that toy or memory.

Not so for Alzheimer's patients. Their *treasure box* gets more and more empty as the disease progresses. They experience the fear of being unable to recall names and faces or to do the things they've done all their lives. The words they've spoken since they began talking are foreign to them, and putting a name to everyday things is a challenge they cannot easily accomplish.

Imagine seeing the fear in a small child's eyes if he were left alone with nothing or no one familiar to him for an hour, a day, a lifetime. This is the fear and confusion that a person with Alzheimer's feels. This fear is with you whether you are alone in a room or at a crowded family gathering... a family they say you are a part of. You are a victim of a disease for which there is no cure.

As the disease begins, the person is unable to recall his memories that have been filed away in the brain, one in front of the other, as papers in a file cabinet, carefully putting each in the order it occurred. The most recent memories are the first files which are unable to be recalled, almost as if they are taken out of the filing cabinet never to be filed again.

The most important—and the first memories (treasures) we have—are love, comfort and safety. Knowing we are answered by our cries of hunger, pain, sickness or fear and feeling the security of another human being, these are the same memories that are the last to go. They actually never leave us and are just more difficult to grasp.

We are by nature dependent on each other from the moment we come into this world until the moment we leave. As you experience your loved one affected by his memory loss, he never loses the need for touch, love, comfort and security. As a matter of fact he craves it, since much of his recognition of everything familiar to him leaves and is eventually gone.

My passion is to care for the elderly, most of all Alzheimer's patients. I am fortunate enough to have seen that, no matter in what stage of the disease, they are always responsive to a soothing voice, a gentle touch and the comfort and love on a daily basis that reassures them — unlike their memory—I am a *treasure* who won't leave them.

My hope for you is not only to enjoy the story of my dad, but also the stories of some of my elder friends, and through these stories may you find something that can help you in life's journey through Alzheimer's or elder care as a whole. When you are faced with a loved one with Alzheimer's or an aging parent, the time spent together will be a *time* in your life, a *treasure* you can put in your own personal files that will hold the most value of all... compassion and love.

Special Thanks

To my loving husband and sons, who without their love and support, I could never have taken all the *time* to spend with my dad.

To my wonderful brother Joe, his wife Debbie and their children, who gave our father a home full of love and laughter, giving Dad the gift of a happy life with Alzheimer's.

To Mom and Dad, for teaching me patience and the value of family.

To God, for giving me the compassion and understanding that I so needed not only to care for my dad, but also to now care for others and help them understand the obstacles of this disease.

And especially to my friend on the farm, who inspired and encouraged me to follow my heart and continue with my book. I will miss her by my side.

I dedicate this book to my dad, the man who though struggling with Alzheimer's disease, gave me the wonderful gift of appreciation and love of others in a manner I never thought possible.

I love and miss you, Dad.

The Journey Begins

My journey as the parent of my parent, my dad, has been an extreme gift to both of us. It seems as though one day I was still his "little girl" and the next day I became the parent, having to make the difficult decisions concerning him—now being the one who would say yes or no, all while feeling that I had the hardest job in the world. Taking on the responsibility of the man I looked up to, respected and counted on all my life... my dad.

He was supposed to make all of the decisions, the unpopular choices and say no when I wanted the answer to be yes. I was the child, not the parent. But now things were going to be different. Now, he would look to me for the knowledge, comfort and security I sought from him my entire life. It was my turn to take on the responsibility of making sure he was safe, to oversee that he ate every day, took his medicine, bathed, changed his clothes daily, etc. It became my job to give him comfort as he struggled to do an everyday activity, to repeat the same things over and over again, until he understood. Now it was time for me to show him the extreme patience and love he had shown me all my life, while giving the answer of "no" when he wanted it to be "yes." The tables were turned. Everything he did for me as my parent now became my job to do for him... I had become the parent of my parent, and life would never be the same.

The scary thing is that much like when your child grows up, it seems as if it happens overnight, as does the regression of a person with Alzheimer's.

One day a small change was the beginning of a road that I- and we- had never traveled, with new challenges every day, every moment. It was bumpy with unpredictable direction at times, but it was a road that became our everyday life and familiar as our daily routine.

My Dad

When my mom was dying, I promised her I would "take care of Dad." Having worked with the elderly at a retirement community and also years ago at a nursing home, I knew I didn't want either of my parents in a facility. I was going to care for them, just as they had cared for me until I was grown— knowing that I needed to be realistic and admit to myself that someday I may have no choice, possibly needing to put Dad in a facility. I also realized at that point it would be something for me to deal with, and Dad would be unaware of the change. I prayed it would never come to that.

Let me first tell you about my dad. He was a handsome, blue-eyed, olive-skinned Irish man. A man with a great sense of humor, who was the life of every party or get-together. He had a way of touching hearts with love and laughter, and you always had a smile on your face when you were with him or even just thinking of him. He would always exclaim, "Are you having fun? Because you know I insist upon it!" And yes, we did have fun; Mom and Dad both showed us how to enjoy life and live it to its fullest.

Dad adored my mom and was a wonderful husband. He was the epitome of the type of husband my sisters and I would wish to marry. Their relationship and love served as a guide to all who knew them as to how wonderful marriage can be.

Though they had been through a lifetime of obstacles, both good and bad, the worst was when Mom was diagnosed with cancer. She made it quite clear she would fight the cancer until it owned her "good days," and then she would stop treatments enjoying what *time* she had and the things she and Dad could still do together.

Tirelessly, Dad cared for Mom while she was sick, and an excellent job he did. She died at home, as she wished, with him by her side of course. Watching them together during her illness and then her death was a whole different level of commitment and love. As their daughter, it was a gift to watch such a beautiful expression of their faith, love and devotion to each other. It was a life lesson for me, a child who was also losing someone very dear- my mom, who I adored- but not my right arm, not my life partner. Dad was lost when she died. His soul mate was gone, and I thought he would never pull out of his loss and depression. But after *time*, he improved and started going out to visit his children. He would come to picnics or crab feasts. It was great to see him "living" again. He even found a companion to go to American Legion dances and out to dinner with. He was as happy as he could be without Mom.

Dad was also a wonderful father, as you will come to see as my journey unfolds. He was a man who was loved by everyone who knew him, both young and old. He was one child in a family of 10, a devoted son and brother, with a twin sister who also had Alzheimer's. He was the father of five children, had 12 grandchildren and three great-grandchildren. Of course, he was the biggest kid of all of us. Mom used to punish him along with us when we were growing up, and later with the grandchildren, because Dad was usually misbehaving too!

Collecting antiques and refinishing them was a hobby of his. He loved to go fishing and crabbing, stop by yard sales or have garage sales of his own. Of course with any money he made, he would treat all of us and our families to crabs and beer to celebrate a good day with his profits. I know by the *time* he did this the garage sale certainly could not have been profitable.

Dad even had a rule where he wouldn't sell any of his antiques to dealers. He would put a sold sign on the admired antique until the dealer left. He would later sell the same antique to a young couple for a good price, knowing they couldn't afford much and would love that particular antique the way he had. The garage sales were actually just a way to talk to people about antiques, fishing and fun and to then have a crab feast with his family!

I always had a good *time* with my dad. Sure, while I was growing up he could be strict at times, but as a parent now, I understand why. He taught me how to love and laugh and to always care about and serve others. But most of all, he taught me to appreciate all you have in life, especially people and family.

My dad loved being at the ocean, bay or reservoir, which were all close to our home. You could see a sense of peace come over him when he was by the water. I remember the day Mom and Dad went to buy their 14-foot runabout (a little crabbing boat). You would have thought it was a yacht. And to them it was. Even now, as I take it out crabbing and fishing, it is a yacht to me also. He and Mom spent endless hours fishing, crabbing and probably necking on that little boat. And on it my sons learned everything they know about fishing, crabbing and the value of *time* spent with their Pop-Pop. Together, they shared laughs, stories and the making of wonderful memories. My family and I will always *treasure* those boating trips; even though the fish were few, the memories were many... that is, before he got sick.

Yes, before he was sick, he was quite a card. Alzheimer's made this a different situation. Oh, he still had the beautiful blue eyes, but they would say, "Don't leave me; I'm still in here." And he still had the olive-colored skin, just aged from the fishing-trip sun.

The one saving grace was when his wonderful sense of humor would shine through giving you a warm feeling that made you realize, it was still Dad. He was still in there. I often thought if he lost his sense of humor, it would upset me more than anything. But I came to know that even if it would only shine through once in a while, the key was to be there when it did and appreciate it.

I realize taking care of someone is not always what we can or even want to do. Not everyone is cut out to give 24-hour care to someone whose health is failing. Whatever *time* you can spend with your parents, then do so because they need you and believe it or not, you need them. The experience will help you grow in a way you would never imagine. It will teach you a level of compassion you never dreamed possible while giving them the sense of love and security that is crucial to an Alzheimer's patient. Much like they made you feel when you were a child and needed reassurance and comfort, it is now *time* for you to give that back. The key to success is to never expect too much, to go with the flow and to be as prepared as possible for... whatever.

Early Signs

Where do I begin?

In the beginning, Dad would call my brother Joe or me and ask how to cook something or question how to operate the washer and dryer. The newspaper would be thrown away, never opened, and the door would be shut but not locked. I began to notice that he had on the same clothes that he'd been wearing two days prior and hadn't shaved since I saw him last.

Now, understand these were things he tended to every day and had done for a couple years after Mom's death. I would check on him at least every other day, as I was concerned about these early signs, and I wanted to make sure he was safe.

Thank goodness before Mom died, she had talked to Dad about power of attorney and to let my brother take care of the bills. Mom and Dad signed everything together, and then filed it with their attorney and doctors. It was so helpful to have all of this in order before he was to a point where he couldn't sign the needed papers.

Joe and I noticed that Dad started to become uneasy or paranoid about certain things. He would tell us things were missing from his house. Actually, he just couldn't remember where he put them. There were numerous times when he felt people were stealing from him, and he even blamed Joe or me. It was hard to witness or be accused of this. After all, we were the ones running up and down the road all hours of the day and night to help Dad. Not to mention, the fact that it was so out of character for Dad. He would have given you the shirt off his back and never questioned it.

The paranoia and fear got to the point where we knew we had to do something. I had read enough about Alzheimer's when Dad's twin sister was diagnosed with it five years earlier to know this was one of the stages he would go through and then move out of. But in the interim, we needed to give Dad a sense of security, and Joe and I needed to get some sleep. The only thing we could do was assure him that we loved him, would never take anything from him and no one else could as the doors were locked. At times, we would blame it on ourselves and say, "Dad, when I cleaned the other day, I must have misplaced it. Don't worry, we will find it again." Sometimes nothing worked, and we received the brunt of the accusations and were asked to leave. Later that day, we might get a phone call saying he had found it or the conversation never came up again. Either way, Joe and I were each other's rock of support, knowing it was the disease and not Dad doing this, while trying not to be hurt. We continued to remind each other and our families that this was not going to be easy.

We Need to Talk

One of the next concerning signs was that Dad couldn't remember how to get to certain places or even recall road names. This was a very obvious change, as his job before retirement was out on the road, and if you needed to get anywhere in our large city, you called Dad and he could tell you three different ways to get there from where you were. At this point, he would only drive to the store or track to walk, both approximately two miles from his home. Grocery shopping is something he gave up quite early, as he found this very difficult. We agreed that I would do the shopping, and I told Dad I welcomed getting out of my chores at home.

At this point even Dad started to notice that he was having problems remembering. He was expressing fear that he was sick and naturally thought of the illness Mom had and the care she needed. (This was a *time* when dementia or Alzheimer's wasn't a household word as it is now. The main concern was cancer.) Dad and I had always had an honest relationship. Therefore, I knew when he questioned me about what was happening to him, he expected me to give him the truth; I did just that. I assured him that he did not have cancer, which was his biggest fear. Instead, he had something called dementia, which in *time* would make it so he would be unable to remember certain things. I saw a look of fear in his eyes, so I hugged him and said, "Don't worry; I will always be with you. When you can't remember, I will remember for you, and I promise you will be okay." Not really sure what he had processed but appreciating the honesty I gave him, I could see in his face that he was relieved and concerned all at the same *time*, and it made my heart ache.

My dad—my rock for my entire life, the friend and buddy who taught me all about life, love and laughter—was relying on me to survive. Not physically but mentally. I knew that day, not only would my life never be the same, but that I would never again be the same person that I was before.

My brother and I sat down with Dad and talked about his wishes, including what he would want to do if down the road he could not take care of himself. Or what to do if he couldn't live alone in the home Mom and Dad had made for our family 50 years ago. He was always very adamant about the fact that he didn't want to be a burden. He wanted to stay in his house as long as possible, but if he had to leave his home, he would like to live with my brother Joe and his family or me and my family. Though Dad's three other children had offered, that was not his preference, for different reasons.

Dad knew he had to talk about this and he couldn't put us off any longer. It was *time* to face that something was wrong. He needed help and was grateful for our love and concern, but not always. Many times he would say, "Don't tell me what to do," or "I don't want to do this." Then he would turn around and say he knew the two of us, our spouses and my sons could not be at his home every second. That day he faced the reality that someday, maybe sooner than we all realized, Dad would have to come to one of our homes. This was probably the hardest reality that my dad ever faced in his life. We assured him he could stay in his home as long as possible, but we needed to make some simple adjustments. He agreed.

I remember the day Joe and I talked to Dad as if it were yesterday. Even though we were adults with families of our own, this was still our dad. Together, we approached him with love but also with fear as to what his reaction would be. We thought, who were we to be telling our dad what he had to do. But united, we continued, knowing it was our responsibility. Much like it had been Dad's when he would approach us as kids for an unpopular conversation.

After we talked to Dad, I realized the hardest thing about having this conversation was not what we would face nor was it the reality of the disease. The hardest part was the look in those beautiful blue eyes that said, "I'm scared and thanks for helping me." Riding home that day was the longest ride of my life because if Dad could have read Joe's or my blue eyes, he would have seen that ours said, "I'm scared too!"

The Plan

Things went well; we had a plan. We knew what Dad wanted, so now we had to keep him safe, happy and in his home as long as possible. We found comfort in knowing what we were going to do when he couldn't stay there alone any longer-he would move in with Joe or me. Weeks that seemed like months went by, with us spending more *time* at Dad's instead of him driving to our homes, as we were concerned about him getting lost, always remembering that it was a delicate situation. He was losing his independence, and we were the ones who had to help him ease into it. I remember saying, "Let me drive; you are retired now, and you should be able to navigate and use someone else's gas money." Always trying to make a joke or let him think he was doing me a favor by making *me* feel needed. Sometimes it worked. Other times he'd get aggravated and would inform me to "stop telling me what to do."

The obstacles became greater, and we would get phone calls from him when he didn't know how to turn the stove off or just that he was scared. Joe or I would go to his home, comfort him and then ride home, knowing we had to do something more to make sure he was safe. At the same *time,* we realized he was not ready to move in with one of us and give up his home, but he also was unable to stay alone.

We Need Help

I began to call him every morning whether I was at home, work or on vacation to check in and to have him take his medication for his thyroid, and then his heart medication after he had a mild heart attack. This would begin to set a routine for him that would prove to be quite important, not only now but also down the road. It too was *time* for Joe and me to realize we needed a routine and, more important, we needed help.

Concerned as to how Dad would handle this, we confronted him with hiring in-home help, trying to make him realize we understood he wanted to stay in his house. But we didn't want to find him after falling down the steps or the house burned down with him in it. In addition, we told him how nice it would be to have the company ("You are such a people person!"). Joe and I tried to keep in mind that it was not about what we wanted to do-but more important, what we knew we had to do. Everything had to be presented in a positive manner, as you would with a child to reassure him. Not that he was a child, but we compared the fear of the unknown to a child with that of an Alzheimer's patient. After all, we had crossed that fine line of being his child to being his caregivers. We had become the parent of our parent.

It was now our continued responsibility to take care of Dad, to keep him safe, and now we knew we could not do it alone. We needed help and we needed it now. Finally, after many phone calls, there were promises from agencies for help and then no one would come. Imagine no one coming to stay with someone who cannot be left alone as you go to work and you don't even get a phone call—what do you do?

We were thankfully referred to a woman (who I will call Mary) through someone at my brother's church. She ended up being the answer to our many prayers. At first, Dad was very hesitant. At times he would even meet Mary at the door and say, "I don't need you to work today; you can go home," at which *time* she would call Joe, who would talk to Dad reassuring him that Mary needed and wanted to be there, while also convincing Dad that he was helping Mary feel useful. This all became so confusing and overwhelming, almost like a game of who can be the most positive! And Joe and I found it to be positively exhausting!

Keeping a Journal or Documentation

We began to write a journal in a simple composition notebook. Whoever spent the day or night with Dad would write dated and timed entries of the activities of the day. This was very helpful in keeping track of his progression with the disease and his daily routine.

Daily routine is probably one of the most important factors, as it would help Dad know what was going to be done on a daily basis. It gave him some sense of security that he could know what he was supposed to do, as best he could, with the continued progression of dementia. It was also very helpful to us so we could keep him on a routine and give him a diversity of people but a stability of daily activities. Certainly, we were not rigid with it but were committed as a team to keep a routine as much as possible. This in turn allowed Dad more independence. Even something as simple as setting the washcloth, razor and shaving cream the same way on the sink, and the repetition of each step every morning.

From this point on, we made a daily record of everything-personal hygiene, what he ate, his bowel and bladder habits, visitors, sleep/nap patterns, if Dad would go for a walk to get exercise, his mood or attitude for that day—it was all documented. I strongly recommend this. It is a priceless tool for the long road ahead. It also helped when we would take him to the doctor. It was our journal of what happened on a daily basis and also how Dad had progressed with the disease since the last visit to the doctor.

It was a wonderful account of daily activities, helping to outline the *time* spent with Dad, not to mention his new likes and dislikes. After all, this was not always our dad who we grew up with-this was our dad with Alzheimer's. Knowing what happened with Dad the day before, or even last week, was very important to give him continuity of care. Not only was it helpful to see when he was troubled about something, but it would also show if he had a good day and why, sparking conversation about that event which would please him and also test his memory. The fact that the documenting gave a perspective from Joe and me along with Mary, our caregiver who wasn't a family member, proved to be invaluable. Mary, a retired RN, was able to give a more objective point of view of Dad's ever-changing ways. (It is harder to face the drastic changes when it is someone that you love.)

Simplify

Motor skills were the next thing to be affected. Dad was unable to figure out how to tie shoes, so we bought Velcro tennis shoes, in both white and black, then he had a dress pair for church. Button shirts were packed away, and pullover sweaters or polo shirts were bought. Many things on the bureau were put away so we wouldn't confuse the daily routine. The belt on his pants, which was really important to him, was always put in his pants prior to giving them to him, so he didn't have to experience the struggle of how to do it. Basically, anything that required a lot of concentration was simplified.

I remember when I would take Dad shopping for these things. We would go together to get him out of the house. I would steer him only to the racks in the stores that had what we needed, and then I held up one item in each hand and asked him which one he wanted. He still got to choose, but the quantities were not overwhelming.

We purchased what we needed, but it was his decision as to which items were bought. I always made sure Dad paid so he would feel like he was buying it, not just standing there realizing he was being taken care of. Then we would go to lunch and celebrate that we had a good *time* and a successful shopping trip.

Dad, being the Irishman that he was, liked his beer. So we would go to this little pub for lunch, where the waitress came to know us. I had long before pulled her aside and informed her that Dad would ask for a Miller but due to his illness to please give him an O'Doul's (non-alcoholic beer). She would come over to the table, address Dad by name, set a frosted mug of non-alcoholic beer in front of him, and he'd smile and say, "My Miller just the way I like it!" Dad never knew the difference. The waitress and I would smile, knowing we made Dad feel like the rest of the vets at the pub. Yes, this took much longer than if I had gone by myself. I could have bought the items for Dad and taken them to him. But he wasn't incapable; he just needed help and patience.

I'll never forget the day we went to Sears for shoes. We had to get shoes at Sears because this was the "best place" to get them, where he had always gone. He needed a pair of tennis shoes as his looked "ratty." We tried on every pair, walking around the aisles of shoes, and finally after about two hours made a decision. They were "perfect!" This *time* I took him home and we enjoyed lunch together. I told him I'd be back tomorrow with my boys to cut the grass. As my sons and I arrived the next day, my dad greeted us as he was coming out of the garage, his heaven on earth. All of his tinkering things were in there. I looked down at my dad's feet and saw the shoes we had purchased only 24 hours ago, looking "rattier" than the old pair.

One of my sons asked, "Where are your new tennis shoes, Pop-Pop?" Dad responded, "These are it—do you like them?"

We all looked at each other, and I asked, "What is on them?" He said, "They looked too clean, so I put some [brown] shoe polish on them and then shined them." At first I wanted to die- all that *time*, all those shoes we looked at. Then I realized this is a man who always polished and shined his shoes for work and church. He never really had tennis shoes, unless he and Mom went out on their little runabout. So, to him, polishing shoes is what you did. He proudly wore those shoes wherever we went. Whenever I looked at them, I smiled, thinking of yet another moment in *time* that I will never forget, knowing this would be a memory to put in my *treasure* box.

So, plan for things to take a long *time*, ignore your watch, notice how grateful they are and be glad you realize the importance of *time* spent together. Something you will often see me refer to is the word *time*. I have come to realize that *time* can be your best friend or your worst enemy. Not only with a sick parent but also through everyday life. People don't take *time* to smell the roses anymore. Everyone is in such a hurry. I, through my dad's Alzheimer's, learned a whole different way of life. A way that makes you appreciate every moment, as you never know how many more moments you have or which ones you'll remember. Embrace the reality that you only have so much *time* left with your parents. So take the *time,* and down the road, you will be grateful. Remember, you will have all of these memories to put into your *treasure* box (your brain) to file away for another day.

If there is one thing I learned in caring for Dad, it is "don't worry!" Make life and situations easier. Get a baby monitor,

only be sure to call it an intercom system or refer to it as "something like a walkie-talkie," never using the word baby. It will give you freedom to go out in the yard or sleep more comfortably.

Simplify daily chores by taking things out of the kitchen cupboards that are not needed on a daily basis, making sure he or she doesn't see you. It seems many elderly people feel as if everyone is stealing from them, even you. Don't lose the trust they have with you. Remember, this is the generation that lived during the war, the Great depression, rationed food stamps, all with one income for large families; they were and are very frugal.

Don't Worry!

Early on, one of the things I found to be very helpful, and most important, is that everything does not always have to be the right way. I will explain this in more detail later.

I remember one day in particular when Dad was at my home for a weekend visit. I was clearing the table after breakfast. Dad was sitting off to the side with my husband, drinking a cup of coffee and watching me. To my surprise, he asked me, "So, have you worked here long?" (At which point I thought, *Okay, he thinks I am the waitress.*) I simply answered "Oh yes, I've worked here forever!" He said, "Well no wonder you do a nice job." I could have corrected him, but why? If he knew I was his daughter, he would not have assumed I was the waitress. Why confuse him more when I could just go with it. In a while when we are doing something else, he'll remember I am his daughter or maybe not. But he knows I am someone who he likes to spend *time* with and he feels loved by—so who cares *who I* am*!*

Something that always stuck in my mind as we watched my dad's memory deteriorate was a conversation he shared with me a long *time* ago. When my mom was dying, my dad said, "You know, I am not afraid to die. I am afraid of the process." I replied, "Dad, that is probably because you have seen Mom suffer so much and for so long" (she was sick with

cancer for three years). Ironically, I look at my dad's Alz-heimer's as a blessing from God. Dad was totally unaware of the process of death. And though he was aware and scared for a short *time* at the onset of his disease, he is now in a happy place, knowing he is surrounded by people who love him.

Don't get me wrong-he went through the defiance, the anger, the determination, the bullheaded days (weeks), but now he is past all that and just happy to be with someone. Someone, anyone, who will take the *time* to spend with him and love him unconditionally whether he has white shoes with brown polish or thinks he has a real beer-he's doing well.

Simple Pleasures

One day, Dad and I were at my house and I had some painting to do. I knew he wanted to help, but I was concerned about the mess it might create. Remembering how important putting polyurethane on his antiques was to him (polyurethane is a liquid that goes on wet but dries clear), I asked him if he would coat my meat block with polyurethane to help protect it. This was an antique I had purchased from him years ago, and it sat on my front porch displaying a beautiful antique pot with flowers. He happily agreed! I poured water into a container telling him it was polyurethane, gave him a paintbrush, and sent him on his way to accomplish a "much-needed chore of mine." When he would get low on polyure-thane (water), I would pour him more. Hours of "hard work" were spent coating my meat block, my split rail fence and my antique pot. He was so proud of the way it looked and how he had been such a "huge help" to me. It warmed my heart to see Dad doing what he loved to do while believing I needed his help. I called my husband and sons instructing them to comment on Dad's accomplishments. When they returned home, Dad proudly showed them the fresh coating of polyurethane to our items. Their reaction made him feel like a million bucks! It cost no money, no mess, only *time*. Mine to be patient with him and Dad to do a job that made him feel useful and still talented with antiques. It was a day that we

ended with pizza and beer while sitting on the front porch watching all the neighbors come home that evening, surely admiring his work as they passed the house.

More Help Needed

As *time* went on Joe and I realized that even though we had help from Mary, we really needed someone to help us with overnights. Until now, one of us had been staying the night with Dad. We rarely had a night both of us could spend home with our families as a whole. We wanted to keep Dad in his house, but we needed another team member added to the mix. Dad had adjusted to Mary coming three days a week, so we thought we would get someone to come three nights a week. Unable to find someone who was devoted, punctual or consistent, we were back to square one. When we had no idea what to do, Joe's friend needed a place to live, and it was a friend that Dad really liked, an old work buddy. This would give Dad a gentleman he could talk to who was not a relative. He would be able to talk about totally different things and stimulate Dad's mind in a very different way. Joe and I talked to Dad, asking him if he would "help Dan out" by letting him live in the clubbed basement. Dad agreed. Now Joe and I would have 24-hour care, and it wouldn't be just our family. It was perfect!

The notebooks were kept up-to-date showing Dad's progression. They warranted the need for another person and we knew it was just a matter of *time* before we would have to adjust things again. But for now we were ok. This worked for about six months before Dad progressed to where we had to, yet again, get a new plan. We started working on making changes at Joe and Debbie's house in anticipation of our next step.

I remember looking in Joe's face and seeing the reflection of my tired face in his, knowing we had a long road ahead of us but also seeing we were both committed to working together, keeping Dad with us and happy. Dad didn't look tired at all!

Moving Out

We made the decision to move Dad in with Joe and his family since his children were small and mine were teenagers. At Joe's, we felt there would be more activities going on to occupy Dad's *time*. Besides, he was always the best Pop-Pop; as I said before, he loves children. As long as he didn't get everyone punished too often, we'd be okay.

In caring for my dad, I have found the importance and value to both an Alzheimer's victim and his caregiver of time needed away from each other. Occasionally, everyone needs their own space or you will drive each other crazy. So we built Dad an apartment at Joe's home in the attached garage. We designed it exactly the same as the first floor in Dad's house only on a smaller scale, which would make his adjustment period much easier. The whole *time* we were building Dad's apartment, he had no idea. We knew if he were aware of the work and *time* that went into it, he would have felt like a burden and would never have moved. Dad just thought Joe was really busy with work.

Moving day was Labor Day, which we circled on the calendar. We showed Dad as it got closer and prepared him for the move. It was very easy to keep him away from Joe's house while we took six weeks to build his apartment. At this point, he didn't have much concept of *time,* and it was summer so we kept him busy until we were ready for moving day. As Joe and I looked around the apartment two days before Labor Day, we proudly thought this would be a great home for Dad. All of the doorways were built exactly the same as Dad's original home to lessen the confusion. We planned to hang all the pictures from his house in the same spots to give it the feel of home. It was intended to look as though we relocated a movie set, and that's exactly how we planned it from the start. We were ready!

When we told Dad it was now *time* to move in with Joe and how wonderful it would be, much to our surprise he was quite excited!

On the day of the move, our sister Liz came in from out of town to assist us with Dad in case he didn't do well. The weather was beautiful. A warm, sunny, summer day-the kind Dad loved so much. Liz kept Dad busy on the back porch, talking about the memories in the home where we grew up and were soon to leave, while reassuring Dad that another family would live here and also make wonderful memories. Joe, our spouses, my sons and I moved everything out. Some things were moved out the back door to where Dad could see them. But most were moved out the front door so it wasn't over-whelming to him. While we said goodbye to the house, Dad smiled and said, "Let's get steamed crabs to take with us and celebrate my new home with Joe!" Joe and I shared a look of a feeling that I will never be able to explain. *Dad was ready.* Ready to move on, ready to be helped and ready to allow us to be the ones to help him. Our sister Liz kept Dad out for about two hours, driving the long way to his new home, past the reservoir. They picked up the steamed crabs and gave us time to prepare. Meanwhile, we hurried to the new apartment to relocate the "movie set" and anxiously await Dad's arrival. I remember Joe and I being so scared, thinking if Dad refused to move, then what would we do?

As we held our breath, Dad entered his new home and his face lit up! He sat in his easy chair looking at the same pictures he had looked at for years and said, "Okay, let's celebrate!" For Dad, this was a crab feast celebration much like we had for St. Patrick's Day or a successful garage sale. But for Joe and me, it was a celebration like no other. It was a celebration of caring for Dad and knowing that though the days, months and years ahead were going to be a struggle with Alzheimer's, today was a celebration of love. A love and devotion that Mom and Dad had taught us and that we were now returning to Dad.

The crabs and beer never tasted as good as they did that day! *Time* had allowed us to create a loving home for Dad, had allowed us to prepare Dad for what was an adventure for him but a new unknown for us. And now *time* was to be spent making sure we never allowed him to look back and want to return to his previous home. This would be where he lived, progressed with Alzheimer's and eventually died, all while we knew we had stood by our promise to be there for him, making sure that he felt safe and loved.

Moving On

After we saw how happy Dad was at Joe's, we knew we had to put Dad's house, our childhood house, up for sale. Though Joe and I were the two youngest of five children, we knew, like everything else, this was up to us. It was as hard as confronting Dad on moving out. This was our house that allowed us to be kids—the house we grew up in, know matter how old you were, you still felt comfort in. It was the home we figured would always be there for us to visit and reminisce in. We had moved all of the furniture out, and the only things remaining were the memories and the remodeling Mom and Dad had done over the years as the family grew.

Putting Dad's house up for sale was easier than we thought it would be. Even though Dad repeatedly would talk about the good times we had there, he also said it was *time* for another family to buy it and have memories there. This train of thought seemed to work for him. With this in mind, we knew it was *time* to sell. We told Dad we would put it on the market, and he never mentioned the house again.

On the other hand Joe and I, came back to the house a couple of nights after the move and pulled lawn chairs and a six pack of beer (real beer, not Dad's O'Doul's) out of our cars. We plugged in the party lights that were a must for any get-together and sat in the family room, where all the parties, celebrations, heart-to-heart talks or sibling fights growing up took place. We sat there talking and laughing at all of the memories and good times that we shared there as a family. Interestingly enough, we couldn't remember anything that wasn't fun or that was negative-we only thought of Mom, Dad, all five of us kids and the great life we all had together. I guess secretly we knew we never wanted to think negatively, at least not out loud, as Dad needed us to be positive in order to help him... we were now the parents.

We sat in the house now emptied of its furniture yet so full of memories, in dim lighting that glistened in the tears that rolled down our cheeks. They were tears of joy for memories made at that house, and also tears of sorrow for the loss of it. They were tears of relief for the easy move and tears of the fear of not knowing what we were facing or if we could do it. But that night, we knew we could mourn the loss of the home we grew up in, reminisce about the good times we had, cry tears of laughter and fear, and then close the door to move on... we were going to do this; there was no turning back.

As I followed Joe out of our childhood home one more *time,* I paused on the steps that I remember helping Mom and Dad retile. For a moment, I saw my dad dancing around the room with me. We danced to the 78-rpm record on the antique Victrola, me standing on his feet, the music getting slower and slower as it needed to be cranked again. I thought, *Well, I guess it is time for Dad to stand on my feet, as I dance him through the rest of his life.*

I left that night with a tear in my eye, a lump in my throat and the knowledge that I would do anything I could to make sure Dad had my feet to stand on and guide him until the day he died. We closed the door, folded our chairs and left. We knew that even though we were brother and sister, we were going to make good parents to Dad, just as he and Mom had made great parents to us.

Time Changes Things

Moving to the next chapter of our journey, in a new home for Dad, we tried to keep our routine normal (whatever that is). We were fortunate that Mary, who went to Dad's old house, now came to his new home and things were going well. The intercom gave everyone freedom to go out in the yard or spend time alone but created a safe environment. The daily logs continued to monitor Dad's progression. Dad was in a home with children, laughter and love to occupy and embrace him. My husband Michael, who had dinner with my dad every Wednesday night at his old house, still came every Wednesday night just as before. My sons, who cut the grass and did chores for Pop-Pop at his old house, came and visited with him just as before. I stayed with Dad three days a week after I changed my work hours to part-time, and I would bring Dad to my house to give my brother and sister-in-law Debbie a much-needed break. My sons would baby-sit the children and stay with Pop-Pop so Joe and Debbie could go out. Everyone was adjusting well and working together.

Then before long, things started progressing rather rapidly. There would be days Dad could not remember any of our names. Recalling the daily routine was a huge obstacle for him. Even recalling what we consider simple bathroom tasks were more than Dad could process. This would create a hectic morning of showers, extra laundry and carpets to shampoo all before 7 a.m. It became more than Joe and Debbie could handle. Mary was doing the best she could, but Dad's Alzheimer's was advancing to the next, more difficult stage, creating even more obstacles. Knowing we could not get help from anyone else and Joe brought in the only income for his family, I had to make a decision.

We decided I would again change my hours at work and help more during the day. This allowed Debbie *time* to tend to her children for sports, schoolwork, piano lessons and other numerous activities. Joe had been taking Dad with him on deliveries for work, but Dad was no longer up to this. So again, the need for adjustment came and together we decided what was best for all. We made sure Dad was unaware of the juggling of schedules, the change to commitments in our lives and the ongoing talks among us to make this work. This new schedule would work for now and allow Dad to remain happy and content as always.

As the seasons changed and the need for adjustments came, we talked among ourselves, changed what we needed to and hoped and prayed for guidance and success for this journey that was such a huge learning experience. The good days gave us hope of Dad getting better, and the bad days that followed brought back the reality of no cure or improvement with this disease. So we took one day, one step, one moment at a *time* and found comfort not only in each other, but also in Dad's contentment, knowing he was surrounded by love. We were in anticipation of the warm days headed our way again, hopeful that summer would help.

To the Beach

Summer was finally here! The ocean always brought such peace to Dad, so a trip to his favorite place seemed in order. This would give everyone a vacation. Joe and Debbie decided to stay home and spend time with their children around the pool while my family and I took Dad to the beach! Everyone was so excited as we packed the car, talking about the smell of the sea air. We rented a place that was right on the ocean, so Dad would not have to make the journey over the dunes. There, he could stay on the deck and enjoy the beauty of the beach he had always loved and shared with us so many times before.

On our third day, Dad's attitude and mood started to change, he seemed uneasy. Though we ate crabs and sat on the deck, both of which he loved, we sensed a fear coming over him. He demanded to go home. This was extremely odd; I could never remember Dad demanding anything. Yet there was no convincing him to stay. We suggested going fishing, but he refused, indicating that he was fearful to go on the boat. (Remember, the boat was where he and Mom spent all their free time.) Even trying to take Dad to his favorite place for dinner proved senseless when he kept his jacket on as if he were afraid to get comfortable. It was time for me to face the realization that Dad needed to go home to his routine.

I explained to my family that I had called Joe and informed him Dad needed to come home. As Dad and I made the three-hour journey, he seemed more relaxed as we got closer. He kept asking me how much farther, just as I had asked him on our family trips as a little girl. As we approached the reservoir by his home, he looked out over the water with the sun beaming down, which made for a breathtaking view. With a loving smile on his face, he turned to me and said, "That is absolutely beautiful. I'd like to take a trip to the ocean. Do you think you could take me sometime soon?" It took everything in me to keep my composure. We had left the ocean not three hours before, after a very stressful three-day vacation of which he wanted no part. Now, he wanted to go to the ocean! I simply said, "Yes, Dad, we will take a trip to the ocean, but not today."

At that moment, I realized more than ever, the unfairness-or perhaps the fairness-of Alzheimer's. It was unfair that he couldn't enjoy the ocean when he was there yet fair because he didn't remember how the trip had stressed him.

That was the last *time* Dad went farther than thirty minutes from home. We knew after this trip it was more than he could handle and more than what we wanted to put him through. He was happy just thinking that someday he was going to go to the ocean again. We were happy knowing that we had at least tried.

After that, Dad and I packed many picnic lunches and, along with Joe and Debbie's children, went to the reservoir for lunch. We enjoyed each other's company, laughed at the children having such fun and I relaxed, knowing that when Dad had enough, it was a ten-minute ride home!

Hats Off

Sometimes things were as simple or as complicated as finding the items that brought security and comfort. In Dad's later years, he wore a baseball cap every day. The more he progressed with Alzheimer's, the more important his hat became to him. The problem was, there were times Dad would take the hat off, unable to recall where he had left it. My sons, who also loved baseball hats, would visit Dad and later say, "When Pop-Pop talks to me, he is looking at my baseball hat instead of my face," thus making them realize it was probably not a good idea to take their hat off around Pop-Pop for fear they would be lost as well! Dad's love of his hat became an obsession, and as a result, we kept hats everywhere. Interestingly enough, at this point of his disease, Dad was never out of our sight for more than a short time. However, we never seemed to find the hats he misplaced. Actually, we still haven't.

One day after much frustration over the fact that Dad would not take a walk, go to the doctor or anywhere for that matter without his hat, I knew I had to do something. After a soccer tournament for my sons, where all the coaches, managers and team helpers wore the same hats, I had an idea. Approaching the gentleman in charge of the tournament, who I knew quite well, I began to be hopeful that I had found a solution to our hat problem. I explained my situation to the coach, which sounded quite comical. And though this had become a huge obstacle for my dad and me, I knew we were dealing with a disease where it could be so much worse. The truth is, all of the small obstacles become large obstacles if you have an appointment and can't find a hat!

Walking away from the soccer fields, my step was a little lighter, my heart a little happier and filled with excitement. I went home to show my family my new purchase-a case of 25 hats! They were the same size, color, emblem, etc. There would never be another lost hat! Thinking I must share these sparingly, I put half of them at my house, a few in my car (just in case) and the others to my brother, making sure I gave one to Dad with excitement in my voice, so he would love it more than the hat he had just misplaced.

From that day on every *time* Dad would say he couldn't find his hat, we would pull one out of our stash and say, "Oh no, here it is," bringing a big smile to Dad and a sigh of clever relief to us.

When Dad died, he was buried in one of those hats. My siblings and I also wore one to make sure we always remembered the importance of the simple pleasures-even something as simple as a hat!

The Rapid Progression

For three years Dad lived with Joe and Debbie. He loved the surroundings, the children and the safety net that went along with being with people who loved him. It wasn't always easy. As a matter of fact, it was quite hard for all of us. Dad needed 24-hour care, and Mary cut back her hours as it had become too much for her. I recall the day Joe and I first met with her. We took her to breakfast and told her what we needed, and she agreed to "help us until we find someone else"—and now, she had been with us for five years. It was impossible to find someone else who would take her place!

It was now becoming more difficult to take Dad out. He needed the comfort of familiar surroundings and his "home base." We would bring activities and visitors to Dad instead of taking him out. And though we wanted to take him to yard/garage sales or out for steamed crabs, we realized it was becoming more stressful for him. He used to enjoy the outings, but those days were gone.

This is one of the hardest things to adjust to. We want our parents to continue to do all the things they used to enjoy, but they are content to have had those times and now have different times. The *time* they spent with friends and family for outings and dances or ball games and travel were wonderful. But their current interests are more about the *time* and who it is spent with, not the event. So take pride in knowing that if you are only sitting on the front porch talking about the antiques you refinished together instead of actually doing it, this is just as meaningful and sometimes more so.

Time (or lack of it) and illness have a way of slowing us down, making us appreciate things differently. You get one chance here; it is not about the material possessions or the title of your job. Though both are important, that is not the legacy you leave behind.

It is more about the treasures in your "treasure box." These are the things you have created and shared with the important people in your life. The stories that will be talked about and passed down for generations yet to come, long after you are gone. Most important, these are the things that make a difference to those left behind.

Our Hospital Visit

One night while I stayed with Dad, he started having severe chest pains. Joe and I were sure it was a heart attack and knew we had to get him to the hospital. The ambulance was called and the three of us went to the hospital, even though Joe and I knew what a traumatic trip it would be for Dad. The doctor told us Dad had suffered a mild heart attack, and tests also indicated evidence of more mini-strokes than he could count. This made sense since Dad's progression of Alzheimer's was more rapid and severe over the last two months. Dad would have to stay in the hospital in the coronary care unit for a few days to be monitored. Joe and I agreed that I would stay, and he would go home to reassure his children that everything was okay.

An easy chair was brought in and Dad and I had a nice, quiet private room. After he fell asleep, I watched the monitors, saw how frail Dad looked and knew *time* would soon become my worst enemy. Dad had gone downhill so much in the past month-could he withstand much more? My prayers were not to pull Dad out of this, but for God to be kind in His decisions for Dad. I felt God had blessed us all along with the strength that we had, not to mention the love and support Joe and I gave each other and also received from our families. Now I wanted God to continue His kindness and let Dad have the dignity we wanted for him. Throughout this deteriorating disease, Dad had his dignity, humor and all the love in the world, all while unaware of the process of death, which he had feared long ago. God had blessed us every day with His presence, and we needed Him more now than ever.

Dad was reassured that I would stay with him and that we would have a "campout" together at the hospital. The nurses loved him, especially his humor and his kind soul. He kept insisting upon taking the Pulsox meter off of his finger. This is the instrument the hospital clamps on your finger which has a red light on it. Dad was so bothered by this and constantly wanted to take it off. So, knowing he had to keep it on, I told him, "When it turns green, you can take it off." I of course new that it never turned green, but as usual I had to think fast and this was the first thing that came to my mind. Luckily, it worked. Dad looked at his finger every 20 minutes and said, "It's still red; I can't take it off yet." I smiled and agreed that we must keep it on. After a while he fell asleep and woke up looked at his finger, made sure it was still red, that I was still there, and then fell back asleep. I found it very odd how he could remember this but not everyday activities-just another mystery in the world of Alzheimer's.

I will never forget long into one night, when I was given the best gift I have ever received in my life. At about 3 a.m., a faint voice called my name: "Trishey." This was my dad's pet name for me. I had not heard him call me that in months. Dad now referred to Joe as the guy who drives the red truck, and he hadn't addressed me as Trishey in ages. Sometimes he used no name or reference at all, as the memory of everyone's name was often gone. Upon hearing him call me this, I immediately thought something was wrong. I even asked, "What's wrong, Dad?" He said, "Do you remember the *time* your mom, myself and all you kids were down the beach and that one huge wave came?" Dad continued with the story recalling every detail, down to the beach where we were, the car we took to get there, and the laughs from the stories told on the drive home.

My mouth dropped to the floor, tears rolled down my cheeks, and for a short *time,* I had my dad back. I again was the child with bright eyes and interest in the love in my Dad's voice, the details he recalled, and the joy of the laughter we again shared recalling that day.

I never took the *time* to turn the light on in his room or to call Joe and tell him to rush over to share this with us. I just drank in every word, and expression, and knew this must have been the sign that I had prayed so hard for, asking for God's kindness for my dad and us as a family. This story and others he recalled, lasted for about 40 minutes, ending with him asking why this thing on his finger still hadn't turned green. I answered with a lump in my throat and a pang of sorrow in my heart at the reality of Alzheimer's "being back." With the shine of fresh tears on my cheeks, I embraced my dad's hand, kissed it, and said, "I don't know Dad, but when it does, I will take it off in a hurry before it turns red again."

Sometimes I wonder if Alzheimer's is hereditary and think it probably is. But I know that no matter how old or sick I might become with Alzheimer's, I will never forget that night with my dad. Just as he loved the water, I too find total peace and tranquility when I am at the ocean. Every *time* I am there, I am reminded of that day—not just the day that Dad was talking about, but more important to me, the day he recalled it. The day he remembered I was his "Trishey" and we had shared a special day with our family at the beach, long ago.

After Dad was stronger, we were moving him to a regular room. Unfortunately, he was agitated, frustrated, and sad that we were not taking him home. Joe and I, knowing that these emotions would escalate the Alzheimer's, talked to the doctor and all agreed at this point that there was nothing the hospital could do that we couldn't do at home. So we quickly packed Dad and his belongings before he was even settled in his new room. We knew the progression of Alzheimer's from the stress would be much worse than what we faced at home in his familiar surroundings. We were going home! Dad, though happy to get home, never got his strength back to where it was before, and we were heading down yet another path of our journey.

Saying Good-bye

I remember, around Thanksgiving, Dad had gotten much worse. It seemed coincidental to think we may lose Dad soon, as we buried Mom eleven years earlier at Christmas time. What a tribute to their love story that he would join her for the holidays. On Christmas Eve, Dad took a turn for the worse and needed a hospital bed for comfort. We knew everyone must have already left work or gone away for the holidays. But as an answer to our prayers and hard work, an angel must have been on our side. Late on Christmas Eve, a doctor who was on call for Dad's doctor wrote the order for the bed and pain medication and said everything was being delivered as we spoke. Miraculously, it was all handled without a glitch, and Dad was able to enjoy Christmas Eve as much as possible in his condition. He had his family around him, telling stories, laughing, and sharing moments together. We knew this *time* was more than precious as it was so obviously limited. Dad never gave any indication that he knew; he just embraced his family. My family and I never even went home to open presents; the only present we wanted was more *time*.

Dad passed away on December 29th with his family by his side, knowing he was going home for New Year's Eve to dance with Mom. He no longer needed my feet to dance on or to carry him. He would be free of pain, free of struggles, and able to dance with the woman who he was meant to spend eternity with.

As I look back, I think, *How did we do this? How did we survive such a hard, overpowering disease?* Then I look at Mom and Dad's pictures and realize we did it because they raised us to work hard, to love with all you have, to take the *time* to care for and love others, and to always be proud of what you do.

I can honestly say I am a different person. The feelings I have when I think of those days, months, and years are not filled with regret, but joy. It was joy from the gift that was given to me of knowing I could make a difference in my dad's life. Just as he did for me, and still does whenever I think of him, which is quite often.

Conclusion

As I recall the last five years, I now see the signs of Dad's failing that we just attributed to "getting older." But now I know differently. The brain has a complicated but interesting quality all at the same *time,* and I hope this story has helped you to recognize some of the stages that I recall. I hope it has helped you prepare for the road ahead and also relax, feel confident, and know you can do a great job. All it takes is love and patience, love and patience, and more love and patience.

I remember the first *time* Dad asked me how to do the laundry (he had been doing it for years while Mom was sick). I didn't think much about the question until he asked three more times that week. Then he asked me to write down step-by-step directions for him to follow. The signs are there—the forgetting of daily things, the change in hygiene habits and the struggle of trying to tie a shoe or zip a zipper.

Many times he'd be mid-sentence and just totally forget what he was saying. *Well, we all do that.* Or, he would forget the names of things or people he was referring to while telling me a story. *I do that too!* So like most people, I would think he was just having a bad day. There were times he called me to come help him with the microwave, and when I arrived at the house, he knew what to do. I often wondered if this could have been his way of asking for a visitor that night. I came to learn that this was the furthest thing from reality. It was my dad's brain closing files that had been available to him for years— files which were carefully placed, one in front of the other. Later, I came to realize that these files would be lost, never to be found or available again.

The best thing you can do is to be patient and start to get a long-term plan in place. Approach any decision with love and compassion but also with a positive attitude. Presentation is everything. If you are okay with the decision, they will follow your lead. Make sure your body language is the same as your words. Alzheimer's patients are forgetful and struggling, but they are not stupid. Give choices when possible, but no more than two options at a time, or it is too overwhelming. Whether it is clothes to wear, places to go, foods to eat or home care versus facility, let them be part of the decision if you can. If they are not able to make these decisions, then you make them and present them in a positive yet firm way. You are the one who needs to be reassuring, patient, confident and strong. Your parents need you just as you needed them growing up. Is it going to be easy? No. Some of the decisions you make will be unpopular. Be strong and positive; in the long run, they will love you for it. You are keeping them safe while also showing them love. That is sometimes the most important thing you can do for someone else. Remember, you have made the decision to take the role of "Parenting Your Parent."

Just as your life changes when you become married or have a child, and then again as you have your next child, life continues to change and get more challenging as everyone gets older. Life with Alzheimer's is like that, only with all of life's chapters in one day. There is no easing into the next stage, no looking up the answers in an encyclopedia or on the computer. You have to make instant decisions, hoping that they are right, and that the reactions you receive are accepted. You need to smile a reassuring smile that says, "Oh yes, this is fine," all the while not having a clue if you are even close to being fine. But you do it, and somehow it works. Maybe not every time, but the beauty of Alzheimer's is that you will get another chance to answer the same question, listen to the same story or solve the same problem. Just as these are repeated, so are your opportunities to answer!

Looking Back

When I look back at my journey with Alzheimer's, I reflect on my "Wonderful Moments in *Time*." *Time* shared by only my dad and me, only my brother and me, and a feeling of joy comes over me for the *time* that we all spent together. We were challenged by a disease that takes you down a different path, a different road, each day, sometimes each minute of every day. The decision of becoming the parent of my dad seems so long ago. I tried to recall when I was the child, the one to take direction and not have a care in the world. I remember always having that comfort zone of knowing I had the reassurance from my dad that everything was going to be okay. You don't even have to be dependent on your parents to have that feeling; it is just a feeling that comes with being their child.

Once my dad died, I felt a sense of loss, as everyone does when someone they love passes away. I knew that just like when my mom passed, I would never be the same person. I would be okay but never the same person. But this *time* it was different. I lost my dad who I cared for every day. I lost the buddy who I looked up to, the man I admired from my earliest memory of our relationship, and the person who I spent every single day with for the last year of his life. The loss was compounded because I was not just his daughter-I was also his caregiver. Now, *time* was my worst enemy. What was I going to do with all of this *time* on my hands? The *time* I had so often longed for.

Reflecting on our "Wonderful Moments in *Time,*" yet knowing I must be realistic of the many obstacles if I am going to help someone else through his or her journey, I recall the early days when Dad was still in his house, the juggling of Joe's and my family's lives. We ran up and down the road to help Dad and reassure him. Sometimes we just gave each other comfort, knowing but not discussing the changes that were happening. I guess subconsciously we thought if we talked about it, then it would become real. We never dreamt that our road would take us where it did. I remember the number of dinners Joe and I missed with our families, the many days we left work to then go and care for Dad until he went to bed. I recall when we needed a break and my oldest son, who was a senior in high school at the time, would go sometimes alone, sometimes with my middle son, to spend the night at Pop-Pop's to keep him company. Then leave in the morning to make the half-hour drive to high school. Dad thought this was so much fun. Having his grandsons spend a weeknight or two with him, how great! Joe and I felt guilty but knew we needed the help. Of course, this led to another obstacle of telling my youngest son that he could not go, as it was a school night. "Why can my brothers go on a school night and not me?" My youngest son would stay on weekend nights with one of his brothers; this lent to more family *time* interrupted and further obstacles. We never dreamt that they would do this for a couple months.

When we were in the very first stages of dementia, I remember telling my sons that they could be involved with Dad's care to any degree they chose. It was their choice, and it was not going to be easy. There would be a lot of sacrifices made as a family. But if they chose to be involved, they would learn a degree of compassion most people don't learn in a lifetime. They all three agreed they would do whatever they could to help me and, more important, to help their Pop- Pop. They did just that.

Before Dad moved in with Joe, I never had the option to sleep in on weekends or vacations. My alarm clock was set to 7 a.m. every day to call Dad and remind him to take his medications, and then I stayed on the phone to be sure that he did. He expected my call. Alzheimer's did not take a vacation so neither could our routine. This was a phone call that I made every day for years. The confusion it would have caused if I didn't was not worth the risk.

For my husband, Wednesday nights were always his night to spend with Dad. No one else-just Michael and Dad. They did this for years. And for some reason Dad never forgot that this was their night. I am fortunate Dad looked at Michael as a son. They had a relationship closer than a lot of blood-related fathers and sons. And no one else dared visit on Wednesday nights, as that was "their *time*." Together, they would have dinner at his house or go to the American Legion. If Dad needed O'Doul's, Michael would take him to a local store to buy it. Even though Michael traveled for his job, he always seemed to be in town on Wednesday nights. Our sons knew if they had a ball game my husband and I would be to every one, unless it was Wednesday night. Then, Michael wouldn't be there. Again, it wasn't worth the risk of throwing off the "routine." Luckily and lovingly, we were all in this together, me and my family and Joe and his family.

The sacrifices for us as a family of five were endless. But the "Moments in *Time*" of love, the bond we shared and the comfort that we gave to each other was priceless. We grew as a family. When most sons are being difficult teens, our sons were helping me with my dad. When most teens are self-absorbed, my teens were helping me.

As I have said before, when Joe and I joined to be the "parents," we had no idea what we were doing. We were fortunate to have a common goal and drive—caring for Dad, keeping him safe and making sure he felt loved. I recall my mom once telling me that "there is enough in life that you can't control, but what you can, you better." This was such excellent advice, and through Dad's Alzheimer's, I reminded myself of that on a daily basis. We could not control Alzheimer's or the progression of it, but I could certainly control how I handled it.

During this time I started reminding my family and myself that "it is what it is." I find myself using that statement on many occasions and also find many of the people I have come to know use it as well. It's a short statement with such powerful words and the meaning to give peace of mind. The phrase itself, more or less, allows you to accept that you cannot change certain things in life. You must accept them at face value. Many caregivers I have worked with over the last few years have been annoyed by my use of this phrase. After a while, they too begin to feel the comfort in these few simple words. It's not that you don't care, just that you care so much you can't let it own you.

Until Dad died, I really didn't notice the sacrifices that we made. We all just felt it was what we set out to do and we did it. I am most proud of my children and the sacrifices that they made-how they embraced the disease and certainly learned a level of compassion that has made them wonderful young men. The last week of my dad's life put this in perspective more than anything.

It was the week of Christmas that my family and I had agreed to put the opening of gifts on hold and spend as much *time* as possible with Dad. This was the first year I did not decorate our house and tree. We as a family decided I needed to be with Pop-Pop, while Joe and his wife needed to keep up their traditions for the sake of their small children. On Christmas Day, we gathered together to a beautiful dinner with all the trimmings sitting at a table surrounded by all of us filled with bittersweet feelings. We were happy to be together finding comfort in our tradition, and very aware that Dad's spot at the table was empty, as he was too weak to get out of bed. The reality of Dad's illness was so very present, not just by the empty spot or Dad in the other room in his hospital bed, but also by the urgency of Michael and my son leaving the table to run to the hospital for a stronger prescription. Trying to be safe in the snow that was falling, all the while feeling that empty sick feeling you get in your gut knowing there is a close end to something you are not ready to lose. We thought even though we have yet another obstacle, it didn't matter—we were still all together. Knowing this would be Dad's last Christmas, we treasured every second not wanting it to end for fear it would be lonelier than what we already felt in our hearts.

My son had planned a trip to go skiing while out of school for the holidays. He spent endless time with Pop-Pop his entire life but knew this particular week might be the last. After being torn as to what to do, he said his good-byes and left for his trip with everyone's blessing, including Pop-Pop's. Three days into his vacation, he received a phone call from me saying Pop-Pop had died. Agreeing that he fly home was a difficult decision on my part. Knowing he had said his good-byes, maybe I should have encouraged him to stay, but then I thought he also needed the closure. I still don't know if I made the right decision and never will but felt there will be other trips for my son, and after all we had been through as a family, I didn't want anyone to have regrets.

As we laid my father to rest, my second parent to die at Christmas time, I once again pulled one of my "treasured memories" from my files. My children were rather young when my mom died and, though upset and sad, still also focused on Santa and presents. I took my young sons to the funeral parlor and explained it like this. "The coffin is the box; the silk lining is the tissue paper; the present is Mom-Mom; and the flowers are the ribbons. We are giving Jesus the very best present we can for His birthday—Mom-Mom." Again, at the same time of year I am burying my dad, now I am giving Jesus and my mom the very best present that we have for New Year's—my dad.

After the funeral on New Year's Eve, we returned to my home and continued with our life, part of which was a party that our sons had long ago planned for them and their friends. My sons said they would contact everyone, telling them not to come. To which I replied, "No, Pop-Pop is celebrating with Mom-Mom, and your friends would have nowhere to go at this late notice." So, we went with our plans, had the traditional New Year's Eve party and realized that this was yet another tribute to my parents showing that family tradition, love, understanding and "Moments in *Time*" were going to continue, just very differently that year.

Yes, life is different... okay, but different. The most valuable part of these changes is that we continue to have every moment make a difference. Thanks to the difficult disease of Alzheimer's, we learned this as a family unit—not just for my family and me, but my brother and his family too.

Where My Journey Has Led Me

The months after my dad's death were very difficult for Joe, myself, our spouses and children. It was a sense of loss that was different from when we lost our mom. It was a gain of *time,* which had been so occupied and busy. Yes, we had plenty to do, but we weren't working around the clock any longer. So we did what we were raised to do: we gathered to celebrate our family, not only in our hearts and souls, but also with our wonderful family traditions. The crabs were bought; the beer was poured; the stories of reminiscing began, as did the tears of joy, sorrow, love and the value of *time* spent together, giving back to a man, our dad, who would drop everything to enjoy the "Moments in *Time*" with his family.

I came to realize I had learned so much about Alzheimer's over the years, and I felt it would be a shame if I did not use it to help others. I was going to do for others what I did for my dad. It was now *time* for me to give meaning, security and stability to as many families and their loved ones as I could. Though it was hard at first, it has become a reward unlike any other. I think of my dad when my clients do certain things and smile, knowing that through him, I learned what to do for them.

It isn't an easy job; however, when I see a beautiful painting, I look with admiration and think, *How can someone paint so well?* Or I may hear a young musician with unbelievable talent, and I am in awe. It is my feeling that, fortunately, we all have our callings—our talents that make a difference in this life. I was not only lucky enough to be given this gift but lucky enough to recognize it.

My gift helped my dad live and die with dignity, never aware of the process of death, as he had been concerned about so long ago. Not to mention the fact that it also allows me to continue to do what I love... to make a difference with other people's *time.*

My Work Continues

In helping others during their own journeys with Alzheimer's, or just their aging parents, I jotted down some of my favorite stories. I hope you learn from reading about the obstacles others have had and how we worked together to overcome them. And sometimes how we just said, "Oh well, there is nothing we can do to change this. Let's just think positive, enjoy and go with the flow."

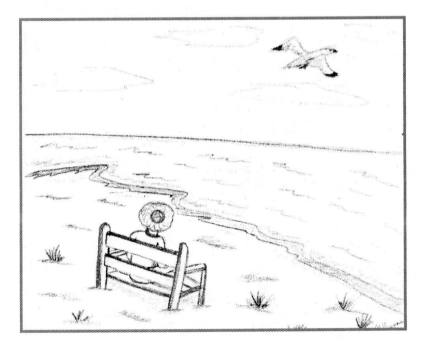

I Can't Sleep in an Empty House

I had been caring for others all my life; now, I was focusing on the elderly who needed someone, whether it was for assistance with a shower, errands or total care. It didn't matter to me... I had found my talent and I was going to use the knowledge and patience that I had gained from Dad's Alzheimer's to give back.

At the *time*, I was caring for four different clients, doing various things, when I received a phone call from a neighbor from long ago. She had numerous health issues over the years; her husband had died, and she wanted to know if I still "cared for others," and if so, could I come and meet with her. Not only was it nice to hear from her, but it was also with someone from my past who needed help-of course I met her.

It saddened me when I arrived to see her sitting in a small condo, decorated beautifully but with no yard. I knew that through all her married years she couldn't have cared less about the house; her beautiful gardens with prize-winning flowers and shapely bushes and trees were her love. But, I knew that would have been too much for her by the crippled hands from arthritis that greeted me when I arrived. So I quickly shifted my thoughts and commented on her beautiful home, decorated with the beauty that only her talents could achieve. We talked, reminisced and then got down to business.

June needed someone to care for her at night. She had a girl for the weekend but needed someone to cover Monday to Thursday from 8 p.m. to 8 a.m. I asked her what she did for care during the days, and she replied, "Oh, I am not afraid to be alone during the daytime!" So now I am looking at my 85-year-old friend from long ago, who has lived through many more challenges and obstacles than I had, and she is afraid to stay in the house alone at night. She continued by telling me, "The biggest problem is that I cannot pay you unless you are a Certified Nursing Assistant, which is how my husband set up our long-term care insurance. The in-home caregiver has to be certified or at least taking the courses to become certified—that is not a problem, is it?" Well, it was a problem; I was not certified nor had I ever even thought about it. I promised June I would check into it and get back to her.

I had met her on a Saturday. By the following Wednesday, I began classes. She was thrilled, and I was in disbelief. I hadn't been in a classroom for well over 25 years. My children were in college. I was too old; what was I thinking? But the next week, I purchased my textbooks, packed bottled water and some protein, which I always told my boys would help them think. Then I drove 45 minutes from my house to school, the only college that still had an open seat in the class, unsure of what I was taking on.

School seemed much more fun than I remembered. High school was as far as I went in my academic endeavors. College was never an option to me. I started work very young, continued working and got married young to my high-school sweetheart. That is what many girls during that *time* did.

College was for the boys or the fortunate girls. So this was very new to me. I loved it!

Not only did I take the Certified Nursing Assistant Course, but I also took a Geriatric Nursing Assistant Course, First Aid, CPR and the Medication Technician Course. The *time* spent with my family was during the days that I didn't attend school. I enjoyed dinner with them and then packed my books, headed to June's home, and after settling her into bed for the night, I would begin a long evening of studies. My sons, who were also in college, would instruct me to "stay focused, no watching TV while doing schoolwork and no missing class." Funny, those words didn't seem as hard to say when I was instructing my boys of these rules.

My family has always been a wonderful support system; it is something that I tried to instill in them, and they learned it well. My *time* was filled with family, school, caring for June and two other clients while knowing that I was doing what God had called me to do; life was full of rewards.

Caring for June continued well after graduation, until she became so ill that she needed to be moved to a nursing home. I look back on that *time* in my life with pride, knowing that I accomplished many things for myself and that I had done it with the help and support of my family. But I was also encouraged by a friend that I thought had moved out of the neighborhood and my life long ago, never dreaming we would cross paths again in such a rewarding way.

I will be grateful to her forever.

Where Am I Going Now?

"A year ago," I witnessed a whole new angle to the obstacles of aging parents. Mrs. Jones, once a resident in an assisted-living facility and now in the progressive care unit, with locked doors and keypads (all of course for her safety), was escorted out of this facility.

Her belongings again were packed up. Her newfound friends left behind as she confusingly moved to a "more accommodating facility." Though I knew it was for her own good, it broke my heart to see the fear and confusion on her face. The family tried to avoid another move by hiring a private duty aide. Unfortunately, the family had "agreed" when they put her in this facility that if her illness progressed to a point where upon she needed care using more than one resident aide or she became disruptive to the others, she would have to go.

But when we as children "agree" to this, we never think it will happen to our parents. They've always been so strong, so self-sufficient. But it does happen. I'll never forget the day she was escorted out, lovingly of course, but nevertheless, turning her back on another place she had called home, another group of friends, none of whom she will ever see again. All she needed was one-on-one care: someone to take the *time* and make the *time*. Again, that ever-haunting word, *time*.

I'm not sure if it broke my heart more to see the family's pain, the employees' pain or the pain of the ones who had become her family (her new friends) who were now left behind. I somehow wonder if in their minds (though often confused) they were wondering, *Will I be next?*

I remember thinking, *There has to be a better way to handle this.* Should the rules permit another floor or unit within the same facility for our loved ones who progress with Alzheimer's more quickly than others? This would allow the availability of familiar faces who could visit daily. Maybe there could be a resident aide assigned to that resident for one or more days a week during the transition, someone to reassure her she will not be constantly moved and, again, have her life turned upside down. Or do we just say we have to do what's best for her (or him) according to the rules?

I don't have the answers. I just know when I would give her one-on-one care, I would take her face in my hands, tell her how much I loved her and that I was glad she was my friend. She didn't yell, didn't fight; she looked at me, not really knowing who I was or what I was doing there, while smiling back not only with her face but also her eyes. That *time* was very well spent and will always be remembered, at least by me. One person can make a difference!

Flowers Always Bring a Smile,
No Matter How They Are Planted

One gentleman I cared for who had been a well-respected professor was now a victim of Parkinson's, numerous strokes and early onset of dementia when I first began caring for him. He lived in his daughter's home with her family and also his wife who was still quite healthy. He was basically confined to his hospital bed. I questioned why he didn't get out of bed. The answer he gave me was that it was too much to get him in and out of bed. When I asked about taking a walk with him in his wheelchair, again the answer was "it's too much." I came to find out that it wasn't too much for him, but too much for his family. To which I replied, "Well, it's not too much for me; I am only here to care for and spend *time* with you."

I proceeded to get him up and sit him in a chair. I made him promise he would not try to get up, and if he did, the neighborhood outing would be called off. He agreed, while smiling at the thought of this adventure he would be part of.

The chair he sat in allowed him to look through the sliding door and inspect the work I was doing to prepare his wheelchair. Obviously this was a chair that long ago had been put in the back of the garage and was now in need of reassembling and a good washing. That way he wouldn't have to share the ride with the many cobwebs that had accumulated.

As I saw him watching me, I found myself also watching him and the new sparkle in his eyes! He had something to look forward to! The excitement in his eyes was priceless to me. When I put him in his wheelchair, I realized he could help me if he took his *time*... again, that ever-so-present word... *time*.

It wasn't that it was too much for his family; it was that he didn't want to be a burden. Our biggest obstacle was that he couldn't keep his leg on the footrest because of his Parkinson's. I asked him if it was all right to lightly secure his leg to the chair with a hand towel. He laughed and said, "Whatever works... I want to go outside." I secured his leg and then covered the towel with his pants leg, so no one could see, allowing him to keep his pride and the uncontrolled leg movements between us.

It was early May and spring was in the air. As we walked through the neighborhood full of beautiful homes, breathtaking trees and a neighborhood that he had not seen for almost nine months, there was a closeness between us. Together, we had accomplished something that he wouldn't let anyone else do. In his eyes, he was not a burden to me, which allowed him to drink in the wonder of the day. I spoke of the beauty of nature, newfound friends and the importance of him getting out of bed and pushing himself to get better. He, with his broken speech from his debilitation, asked me to lean down to him. I stopped next to his wheelchair, stooped down next to his legs, which were shaking from his disease. He spoke to me, his words slow and difficult to express, a small tear in his eye, looking so serious and overjoyed at the same *time*, saying, "I want you to know I will etch the memory of this day in my mind forever." To which I replied, "And so will I. It is a perfect day."

After our walk, I wheeled him to the back of his home and fixed us a picnic lunch to be eaten by the pond. The pond was built for him as a reminder of his own home in Virginia, a pond that he had never seen as he had been too sick. We sat sometimes talking, sometimes just drinking in the beauty of friendship and the simple pleasures of making a difference.

Over the next couple weeks of caring for Professor David, I came to realize he loved gardening. However, with his health, that was impossible-or was it? After one of our daily walks, I told him I had a surprise for him. I spread plastic over the picnic table, took pots, soil and small flowers to be planted out of my car and put them on the table. As I started to put a pair of gardening gloves on his shaking hands, he said, "No, I want to feel the dirt." I watched him turn the soil over and over in his hands. What would have taken a half hour for either you or me took him the entire day. Perhaps it was because of his disabilities or perhaps because he so enjoyed it-or maybe the combination- I'm not quite sure. He repotted the flowers and ate lunch at the same table, refusing to move (maybe for fear he wouldn't be able to finish or because this joy would end too soon). As he was enjoying his lunch, I had him direct me where the potted plants should be set around the garden and deck. He directed me and then redirected me until they were perfectly placed, sipping iced tea, admiring his job well done, all while glancing to his pond and back to his flowers.

I only cared for Professor David for a few weeks while his wife was out of town. I keep in touch, sometimes visiting him and his family. His dementia has progressed; he is still debilitated from the Parkinson's, but he is now up and dressed every day. He is wheeled through his neighborhood, no longer needing to have his leg secured. I am told he has repotted those original flowers (and many more), which he gives away to anyone who visits.

I did nothing but make him feel useful, capable and part of the family, not a burden. The initial reaction when someone has such health problems is to keep him (or her) in a chair or bed where he is safe. What we must realize is that if one's mind is happy, it can help heal the body.

It is crucial to figure out a way to let our parents enjoy their hobbies. If Professor David can't get down to the garden, then we should bring it up to him. The results are priceless "treasures."

Teaching an Irish Girl
Italian Traditions

I received a call one day from a woman who needed help with her mom. When I arrived, I found a thin, frail 94-year-old Italian woman with the spunk of an 18-year-old. She was very hard of hearing, able only to get around with a walker and insisted she didn't need care (which is typical). But she was showing signs of dementia and certainly couldn't be left alone. Because she claimed she didn't need any help, I ran into much resistance. But through patience and persistence on my part, we became very good friends and she looked forward, as did I, to the *time* we spent together.

I learned that she loved to crochet, do crossword puzzles and play card games, none of which were played by the rules. Of course, she took many catnaps during the day (it is tiring being 94). She spent most of her day on the sofa with her feet propped up and a blanket tucked tightly around her, as she was always cold. Therefore, I had to be creative with what we did together, since it all had to be done on the sofa. I pulled out her photo albums (after getting her permission, of course). Unsure if it was a good idea, I asked her who certain people were. If she knew someone, she would go on and on with stories about them or the memories she shared with them from times gone by. The pictures she didn't recognize, I would simply tell her,

"They must be friends of your daughters."

It gave her a sense of security that she could remember certain things and people and that she had a captive audience in me. On other days we would sit and crochet-she had the job of holding the yarn on her hands and instructing me on how to "do it right." We would put a TV tray on the sofa between us and play go fish, pinochle, bridge and rummy all at the same *time*, with me following her lead, as she knew the rules and somehow she always won. Go figure.

Sometimes she would be adamant about why I needed to be with her and why I wasn't at work like everyone else, to which I replied, "I have off today and I wanted to come visit." If she didn't want me there, I would busy myself in the kitchen or take towels and washcloths out of the closet, put them in a basket and ask her to help by folding them.

I'll never forget the day when she asked me where I worked, knowing all the *time* that she was wondering why I was never at work and when, if ever, did I work? I explained that I worked for my brother's concession business as a bookkeeper (which I did part time). She said, "Oh, he's a councilman; you must be so proud." I said, "Oh yes, I am very proud."

I could have corrected her and said, "No, a concession business, not councilman," but what's the point? That wasn't what was important. So I just went with what she thought and never felt there was a reason to do any differently.

When she continued to ask why I was there or say that she didn't need anyone with her, I always tried to change the subject and proceed to make her feel needed. I would take a magazine and ask her if I could sit on the sofa with her. She'd reply, "Yes, but I am not looking at that magazine." Before long, she was peeking over at the pages and commenting on different pictures.

The key to all of the things we did together was that she did them in her own *time* and in her own way. It was the one independence that she still had control over. I would comment on how much I learned from her, always keeping things positive.

The best memory I have was of the day we made pizzelles. I am an Irish girl, so I had no idea what these were and certainly did not know how to make them. But it was Christmastime and an Italian tradition of hers to make them as gifts for the neighbors. I asked her daughter to make the dough, and the next day we set up the pizzelle maker (which is much like a waffle iron), the dough, powdered sugar, etc. That day I was taught by my newfound friend the proper way to make this pastry that she had made all her life. Only now with her dementia it was a task that took much thought, since it was a routine that had to be done in exact, repeated steps. But she did it; she made them "by herself," showing me every step over and over. She beamed with excitement as she dipped the batter on the griddle, checking them a million times until they were "just right." Then I was allowed to sprinkle the powdered sugar on them. It was a lot of pressure on me, after she mentioned, "I guess you could do that step without doing it wrong." Of course, I was instructed to "not put too much or too little sugar as it would ruin the taste." What probably would have taken one hour took four. But it was a lifetime of happiness to me and a day that she spoke of until the day she died. I will always think of her when I hear the name pizzelle and cherish the fact that a woman of 94 could still make her wonderful Italian pastry. She taught me, an Irish girl, exactly how to do it, "the right way." No matter how old you are, you still have so much to give, if only someone takes the *time* to listen and learn!

Don't Turn Off the Ball Game

A very dear friend of mine moved herself and her family in with her mom, Sue, after she had become advanced with dementia. Sue was a huge baseball fan who would watch professional baseball until the game was over. Nine innings or twelve, 10 p.m. or 2 a.m., it didn't matter. She couldn't remember her own name, her children's names and certainly not her grandchildren's. But she knew all the players' names (of course just the ones on her home team): "They are the only ones that matter."

Sue's biggest obstacle was that she couldn't remember how to do daily activities. The everyday things she did for years were now forgotten or too much effort. Therefore, it was always a verbal battle to get her in the shower, to have her eat meals or come out of her TV room. After all, "The game might be on." This meant she would not come out of her room until the news was on, which is how she knew it was not game time.

It was my mission to help the family to get Sue out of her TV room to interact with others, thus slowing the progression of her dementia by keeping her stimulated.

Sue lived in a house near a body of water that had been her home where she raised her children and grandchildren. There were beautiful sunsets, birds and boats. All of the things she would rush outside to enjoy her entire life were now the last things she wanted to do. We felt she not only needed the fresh air but also certainly exercise. (Exercise and range of motion are so important to maintain and promote mobility.) How do you incorporate all of that with baseball?

We set up a comfortable chair on the back deck, along with a glass of juice with a straw, just as she liked it, and a TV. Now we had baseball, sunsets, birds, boats, juice, fresh air and the exercise to walk to the deck. Sue was thrilled and so were we.

As Sue's Alzheimer's progressed and the baseball season ended, we continued to go outside on the deck and enjoy nature, which was so much a part of her past. But she never held many conversations that didn't include the people she remembered most: her ballplayers. The stimulation of the additional activities that she could witness and the conversations she could join in when she wanted to made a huge difference in her mental status. This enabled us to get her bathed and dressed before she would go out on the deck. It wasn't everyday, but we just learned to pick and choose our battles if we were going to get her up and out... who cared if it was in her bathrobe?

We learned a valuable lesson in adjusting our everyday life to make everyone happy! And occasionally we put in one of the taped ballgames to get us through a long night (knowing it didn't matter if it was baseball season)—at Sue's house, it was always baseball season.

Fishing Trip Gone Bad

During a *time* when I worked at a facility specializing in Alzheimer's, I learned something very important. The most valuable gifts you can give an Alzheimer's person is patience, understanding and withholding judgment on his or her perception of things, whether it be right or wrong by our everyday standards.

Early one morning as I walked into the facility, I was greeted by one of my residents already troubled by something he didn't know how to handle. He urgently motioned to me, waving his arm as if he were in pain, indicating that I needed to drop everything and tend to him, which I did. My purse still in hand, my jacket on, I sat on the arm of his chair, asking him what was wrong.

He proceeded to show me the top of his hand and tell me, "I can't get the fishing hook out." I looked at his hand, and obviously, there wasn't a fishing hook. I asked if he meant the veins (which showed so prominently in his aged hand). He said, "No, I see those veins, but don't you see the fishing hook in my hand next to the veins?" To him, this was very real and quite concerning. So I knew if I was going to help him and he was going to trust me I too needed to believe the hook was there. So I asked him how he got the hook stuck in his hand. He proceeded to tell me, "I had 15 fishing hooks and didn't want anyone to get hurt. So I stuck them in my pocket, then I reached in to get something, forgot about them and got this one stuck in my hand." His biggest fear was that he would have to go to the hospital to remove the hook if I couldn't help him. I assured him I could and would take care of him.

Trying to think fast, I reminded him of the wonderful remedies of long ago known as drawing salves. I told him I would put this on his hand and it would draw the hook out. It would probably happen when he was sleeping and not moving his hand. I explained that I would put this salve on and it would draw it from his skin. He was greatly relieved and assured that this was the best way. Knowing there was no hook, I intended to use a generic hand cream, but also didn't want him to see the container for fear he would see it wasn't drawing salve. Therefore, I put the regular hand cream in my palm and went over to him, rubbing it on the top of his hand, as he watched with hopeful, loving eyes. He patted me on the hand and thanked me for taking such good care of him.

As I looked over at him throughout the day, he would be looking at his hand to see if the hook was still there. For three days, four times a day, cream was put on the top of his hand. Miraculously, the hook was never mentioned after the third day and it was never "seen" again. I learned a valuable lesson, which I will never forget—just because something isn't real to you does not mean it isn't real and therefore worrisome to someone else.

Trusting someone to help you is a wonderful feeling!

Don't Forget the Horses
Need to Go In

The opportunity to care for Lance, a gentleman who had previously owned prize-winning horses, was a wonderful experience. His room was decorated with all of his ribbons and photo's. The facility where I cared for him was coincidently in the country with a horse farm across the field. Originally a city girl, I was fascinated by his stories of horses, jockeys, races and the thrill of the victories. He was fascinated with such a captive audience. He suffered from Alzheimer's, and though he couldn't remember how to tie his shoes or cut his food, he could recall every detail about his racehorses and those exciting racing days.

One day, the clouds moved in and the sky became dark; a storm was heading our way. I noticed Lance getting uneasy in his chair. Then it dawned on me-the horses! Lance suffered from sun-downing, and a storm at 5 o'clock in the afternoon only made it worse. (*Sun-downing is a marked increase in agitation and confusion in the late afternoon and evening.*) I went over to him and told him I had called down to the barn and had the farm hands bring all the horses in before the storm. His shoulders relaxed; he sat back in his chair and thanked me profusely.

That day I learned the importance of being in tune with anyone you care for. I thought back to when my children were young and I knew all of their fears or worries. Now I realized that if I was going to do my job to the best of my ability and help my patients cope with the brutal disease of Alzheimer's, I would have to be in tune with them in the same way. Everyone I have shared this story with has asked me, "How did you know to tell Lance that you got the horses in the barn, when really there were no horses at all?" I simply replied, "To Lance there was, and it was my job to know that and respond."

After that day, when ever a storm headed our way, I would close the windows, turn on the lights and inform Lance that the horses (that really didn't exist) were already in the barn! Coincidentally, the day Lance died, the window in his room was cracked open. I prepared him for his family to come and say their final good-byes. The room was peaceful enough to hear a pin drop. Off in the distance, I heard a horse from a neighbor's farm whinny. I knew Lance was being called home. He was going to ride home in style.

Through Lance, I learned the importance of knowing the backgrounds of the people you are caring for and how to give them comfort before the fear they are experiencing becomes worrisome.

A Nice Day Out with the Family

Once, I had the pleasure of working for a couple that decided to take residence at a retirement community. This lovely couple had been married 52 years. Unfortunately, both had Alzheimer's.

When I first started caring for Bob and Sally, they were at different stages of the disease. He was unable to feed, dress and bathe himself, and she only needed help bathing and assistance with the other duties. They shared the same bed, looked at each other with loving eyes and stayed next to each other 24/7, as if they were afraid to be out of each other's sight, for fear that something would happen. She was able to hold a conversation, even though she didn't always make sense, and he understood but rarely responded. I watched them together as if there was a bond, an understanding with no words spoken. I guess it's one of the many gifts you have together after being married so long.

Over *time*, Bob had progressed with his disease to where he was failing and bedridden after numerous other health issues. Sally really didn't understand what was happening to Bob. Her Alzheimer's had progressed to a degree where she would ask about Bob, but if she didn't see him, it was okay.

The day Bob died, Sally was unable to process what was going on. Their sons took her to the funeral, brought her back with a folded flag in her arms and flowers to decorate the house. She said she had a "nice time" on her outing with her family. This was a reality to all of us that cared for them as to how brutal, yet kind Alzheimer's could be. Brutal, because she had no idea her husband had died. Kind, because she had no idea her husband had died. Rather bittersweet. Whenever she asked where Bob was, I would say, "He is at the hardware store," or other times, "Out fishing with your son." She would always reply, "Oh good, Bob likes that. I'm glad they didn't ask me; I wouldn't have wanted to go." I learned from Bob and Sally the devotion of a wonderful marriage of 52 years. But I also learned that with this cruel disease, there is also a kinder side. I can't imagine being married for 52 years and then living without the love of my life.

Whether the disease would not allow her to realize that Bob had died, or the pain of losing him would not allow her to face it, it didn't matter. My job was to keep her happy, safe, loved and by no means longing for him.

I would never know the feeling Sally truly had. But what I did know is that… how things appear through our vision is not always how they are felt through someone else's heart.

Give Me the Bill

Our parents' and grandparents' generations were and still are concerned about paying their own way. Many lived through the depression and know the value of the dollar and homeownership, better known to them as the "American Dream." Thus they never want to owe anyone anything.

Though I have seen this often, it became most prevalent to me when I worked in a retirement community many years ago. One couple in particular comes to my mind. Everything they ate, services of laundry, entertainment and all they needed to live were included in one price. Their son, who had the power of attorney, paid this monthly fee. There was never a question or concern except at mealtime. Dinner would be served and Nellie, sitting at the table with her purse on her lap, would tell her husband not to eat anything until they knew how much it cost. Trying to reassure them that the meals were free was not acceptable. And they certainly would not understand that it was included in their fee. They believed it was kind of me to allow them to live in my "huge home." By no means would they agree to eat my food also. So every night it was the same obstacle. I found it funny that this refusal never happened at any other meal. (I guess Nellie and Tim went out to dinner quite often in their younger years.)

One night, when this became a reason for them to refuse dinner, I decided to charge them $2 for the meal. Happily, Nellie paid the $2 and said she thought the prices were so reasonable, they would surely be back every night! I instructed the other employees to always take the $2 so Nellie and Tim were "paying their way." Later, when Nellie would go to bed, she would place her purse carefully in the closet. The staff was instructed to replace the $2 in her purse for the next evening. Night after night, Nellie and Tim would proudly sit together at dinner. Nellie would complain that Tim never had any money, and she would pay the same $2 each night, showing that she would never take advantage of my kindness in having them for dinner. I laughed while thinking, *I wish my money would stretch as far as Nellie's, or more important, I wish I could find a place to enjoy a wonderful dinner for $2!*

Make Sure Everyone Will Be Okay

Not knowing where I would get my next client was never a worry for me. Somehow, it always just seemed to happen. When one of my clients would pass away or be moved to a nursing home, I would get a call from someone else who needed me for a family member or friend. Trust me, there are so many people who need assistance, which leads me to the story of a dear friend of mine.

Nanny was a neighbor of mine for 22 years. She was a tough woman who raised two sons on her own back when that was unheard of. No matter how bad the marriage was, you didn't divorce-you stayed together "for the children." Not Nanny. She wanted more for her and her sons. She got just that. Her children were grown and moved out on their own. She not only showed them how to love and laugh but how to appreciate the little things in life and the value of devotion to what is important.

When she became ill (being the tough cookie that she was), she did for herself for quite a while until one day her son said, "No more, I am moving back home to care for you the way you have cared for everyone else all your life." Caring for her and taking *time* for her was nothing new to him. The two of them had taken vacations, cruises and outings together for a long *time*. They were more than mom and son; they were best friends. There was a mutual respect of what Nanny had done for him and what he was going to now do for her.

Again, the feelings of *time* with my dad had come to the forefront of my career. The reality of the pain my friend would experience, as Nanny's son who was going through many of the same emotions I had years ago, brought a sense of compassion to me that was very different this *time*. He was not facing the Alzheimer's as I had since her problems were more physical. But he was certainly facing the decisions of parenting a parent who was always so strong and independent. He was going to have a tough road, and I was going to help him in any way possible.

When I was walking in the neighborhood one day with my husband, a voice called to me from my neighbor's porch: "When you get back from your walk, I want to talk to you." It was Nanny; though she had a given name, everyone who knew her called her Nanny. As promised, I stopped on my way home and Nanny had asked if I would come by and give her a shower two or three times a week. She said, "My son is doing a great job in helping me, but I would like you to do this if you don't mind." I agreed with the understanding that if when I came she didn't feel up to it, she would tell me and I would come later that day.

For months, I would greet her in the morning to shower her, telling stories, laughing and sometimes just reassuring her that her family would be okay when she was gone. That is one gift that I have given everyone who I have ever cared for—

honesty. I have never sugarcoated anything. I have always answered questions about my feelings of life after death, the reality of their illness, the beauty of the gift of family and memories kept forever in their loved ones' hearts.

Throughout Nanny's illness, I had the pleasure of seeing her son care for her day in and day out. The amount of love that showered her was not only from her sons, but also from her niece, grandsons and friends from long ago or newly met. She was a tough woman who was not only a survivor herself, but who also taught others how to survive by her actions, her words and her tireless stories of what matters. What mattered most to her now was that everyone would be okay when she was gone.

My *time* spent with her had increased from showering to visiting, reading with her, talking about her beautiful dollhouses and the *time* and love that went in to decorating them. Not to mention the beauty of friendship, motherhood, sons and the things she needed to do before she "went home."

Our showers turned into bed baths, as she was too weak to make it to the bathtub, which was hard for her to accept—not because she was upset that she was too weak, but because she had another neighbor remodel that bathroom years ago. She was so proud of the choices that she had made of colors, tile and the bars for safety, that she was upset to not be able to see it every day. I laugh as I now retell this story, remembering when I asked Nanny if she wanted me to take a picture of the bathroom so she could hold the picture while I gave her a bed bath.

We laughed a lot, Nanny and me; she gave me a gift of strength and a different outlook of survival like no one had before. In the last month of her life, I spent *time* with her almost every day. We were lucky; I could walk to her house any *time* day or night. Reassuring her that her *time* was coming (as she was getting quite impatient), she asked, "What is God waiting for? Doesn't He know I am done?" Many nights I would sit with her son, both of us in disbelief that she was still "hanging on." She became known as the "Tireless Rabbit" and that is what she was called. A name that she was quite proud of! We found a stuffed rabbit that fit the part of such a name and gave it to her. Nanny proudly displayed this on her dresser and was laid out with it when she died (on Thanksgiving Day).

The night before she died, I had the honor of spending *time* with her and her son. I left late that night, knowing that my dear friend would be called home for Thanksgiving.

Somehow, I think the day she died was a message to all who knew and loved her. She was so very thankful for all she did, all she had and for the love of family and friends. Oh, don't get me wrong; she was that tough cookie right up until she died—the tough cookie that survived many obstacles in her life and was open and honest with her feelings, good or bad. You always knew where you stood with her, and that is rare nowadays. I thankfully had the pleasure of knowing and serving my very dear friend. Every Thanksgiving Day, I say a special little prayer to her as one of the people I am truly thankful for having had in my life, our "Tireless Rabbit."

Happy Hour Continues

As we get involved in our lives, we forget that the elderly used to do the same things we are doing now. They were CEOs, accountants, horse breeders and parents—all as we now are. Yes, they have gray hair, wrinkles and maybe a forgetful mind. But, it is still the woman who once was a little girl who giggled at silly things and told stories at slumber parties with her friends. Or it's the boy who climbed trees, collected baseball cards or played ball in the field, hoping to make the winning run at home plate. The elders of our lifetime still have these feelings, the unconditional love of people and moments. The difference is, they are dependent on us to help them relive these moments.

This came to the forefront of my reality when I worked for elders in a facility. While having a group come to entertain with music, one of the residents said, "This is a great happy hour, but where are the drinks?" I never dreamt that happy hour would come to mind for 80- and 90-year-old people. Thinking this through, I realized this was the generation that would go to the VFW or the officers' club many years before. Therefore, in order to remedy this request, I bought a blender, made virgin daiquiris, watered down the wine for the ones still allowed to drink and brought that (ever so helpful) O'Doul's for the beer lovers.

Together, we would dance, sing, drink and celebrate Friday happy hour with the love of our social *time*, good friends and of memories I thought didn't exist. The only difference from that happy hour, and the kind I attend with my friends, is that the happy hour with the elderly must start at 3 p.m. to be sure bedtime will still be 7 p.m. as usual! Through our Friday happy hours, I also realized not to judge by the shell of a person. They might be elderly, but the young habits of long ago still make us who we are, reminding me once again, "I'm still in here."

Our Grocery-Store Adventure

Not so long ago, I cared for a gentleman who tried very hard to maintain care for his wife and the home they had shared for their 50 years of marriage.

His inability to face the reality of his advancing dementia, or the need for help, led his family to decide to have me come and be a companion to him. This allowed me to oversee his nutrition along with keeping him as active as possible for as long as possible.

To accomplish these goals, I would spend three days a week, from 8 a.m. to 4 p.m., thus overseeing two meals. His family would take care of the third meal and the other days.

Our *time* together was exciting and full. Vince loved to be outside and loved taking adventures in the car even more. Since he long ago stopped driving, he was ready to "go out" the moment I would walk in the door.

The day began with him insisting on a good breakfast. Knowing he would then be able to go out with me encouraged him to eat and "get that over with." Unfortunately, eating good meals is not a priority to people with dementia/Alzheimer's Simply, they not only forget how to prepare certain foods, they also don't always remember each meal. Quite often, they look at the *time* of day and are sure they must have already eaten.

After breakfast, we would take a walk in the neighborhood while engaging in conversation about everything and anything. Of course, we carried a pocketful of dog treats for the dogs in the neighborhood that would join us along the way. This was the routine that we kept every *time* we were together, except for rainy days when we would go to the mall and walk there. Riding out of the neighborhood we would be sure to throw a dog treat out the car window every couple feet to let the dogs know we hadn't forgotten them when they came outside to "do their business." I used to tell Vince, "I feel like we have a paper route, only with dog treats!"

Vince and I would take long rides whenever the weather allowed. At each intersection, I would ask him which way to turn. He would get a big grin on his face and say left or right. At which *time* I made a mental note to myself, so I knew how to make our journey home at the end of the day.

On Wednesday we would take a short ride and then make our way to the grocery store, just as he had done for all of his retired years. The store list would be written and added to throughout the week. This adventure would begin with Vince happily getting the cart and inspecting the list so he knew where to begin.

When I first started caring for Vince, he could do the shopping on his own, relying on me only for transportation. Now it was different. Vince could not figure out how to push the cart and find the items on the list at the same time. It took him great effort to remember and achieve the steps of grocery shopping that had come so easily to him not so long ago. I found the best way to handle this was to guide the cart to the section for one item at a time. Discretely, I would point him in the direction of where I thought the item might be and patiently wait while he read every label, rechecking the list to remind him of what he was looking for. Upon finding that particular item, he proudly handed it to me with a great sense of accomplishment and pride. We then proceeded to the next item on the list and began the same process of searching again. The task of grocery shopping took a great deal of *time,* patience and persistence. Our last item placed in the cart was a candy bar for Vince to celebrate a job well done!

Vince died after a long battle with heart problems and Alzheimer's. He left behind a wonderful family and a new perspective for me on grocery shopping. As I walk through a new grocery store, frustrated at not being able to find the items I want, I think of Vince and smile, knowing that I need to conjure the same persistence and determination to accomplish my list and then treat myself to a candy bar!

Bringing Home the Beach

Though I have cared for so many people throughout my life and each one holds a special place in my heart, I have to say the next story is one of my favorites. This particular woman held the same love of the beach as I do, and I could understand her need to go, one more *time*. The problem was, she was not strong enough to make the trip. I, on the other hand, was planning a week's vacation to the beach, and I promised I would bring it back to her. I did just that.

As my husband and I were packing the car to head home after a relaxing vacation, I, true to my promise, had a couple things left to do before our journey home. I needed to bring the beach home to Elizabeth!

The suitcases were packed, the bikes were tied onto the car and the bucket in my hand, I headed down to the beach for my supplies. While filling the bucket with sand and making sure I had enough, I finished drinking the water bottle I had. This would need to be empty so I could fill it with ocean water. One last stop and we were headed home. The fudge store didn't open early, so we leisurely left town to be sure to get the final item that I needed.

Tomorrow, I would deliver the beach to my friend who had the same love as I did for the wonderful sun, surf and sand.

The love she got from her dad, just as I had from mine, many years ago. I couldn't wait to get home. It was the first time I could ever remember not being upset that I was leaving the beach. But I was on a mission. My 91-year-old friend needed to have a beach fix and was counting on me to deliver it.

Monday morning came and I hurried over to her house. The sand was dumped in a wide basin, then set outside to be warmed in the morning sun. The ocean water was transferred to a spray bottle and the CD of ocean sounds, with the cracking of waves and squawking of seagulls, was put into the CD player. Suntan lotion with the scent of cocoa butter was poured on the patio table. Now all I needed was Elizabeth to wake up. I was going to take her to the beach!

Two hours after the beach was set up, Elizabeth and I headed outside to the patio. I pushed her in her wheelchair, having her close her eyes, instructing her not to peek, or it would ruin the surprise. Unsure of what I had planned, she giggled with excitement, forgetting that a week ago I had promised to bring the beach home to her. As I pulled her over to the suntan-lotion–soaked table, I reminded her first to keep her eyes closed, to lift her feet (allowing me to direct them into the warmed sand). Pushing the play button on the CD player, the surf and seagulls were music to her ears. I spritzed her with the ocean water and took her hand, placing it into the bucket containing the remainder of the sand. She squealed with excitement, saying, "I can't believe you brought the beach to me, just as you promised!"

Together, we sat with our eyes closed, listening to the ocean, smelling the beach and sifting the sand through our toes. For lunch we ate the fudge first and then our sandwich, making it a true beach experience of a typical vacation where you break the everyday rules of how things are supposed to be.

Elizabeth relived that day every day for a week, saying, "I do not want one day at the beach—I want an entire week, just like I had when I was a kid!"

All my life, the beach has been the place I have loved more than anywhere else. My dad and mom were the same. Elizabeth and her parents were the same. This particular week's vacation, both at the beach with my husband and again with Elizabeth on her patio beach, reminded me of the lucid conversation my dad had with me when he was in the hospital.

I hope and pray that if I forget things in my life, the beach and the times spent there will not be among the memories lost.

I also hope that when I am 91, someone will bring the beach to me and spend a week on my patio, pretending it is the true beach. If I too am unable to go to the beach, I want the beach to come home to me!

Accentuate the Positive

The opportunity came to me to care for a gentleman that will always come to my mind when I listen to the song "Ac-Cent-Tchu-Ate the Positive." We shared the same love of music and would sit in his beautifully decorated home that he and his wife still shared for their soon-to-be 48-year marriage. His wife enjoyed music but preferred the quiet sounds of the birds in their garden. So when his wife would take a nap, Jack and I would put in the CDs I had purchased of his beloved artist, Johnny Mercer, and we would sing at the top of our lungs. I found such pleasure in these times together, as he really knew how to do just what the song said: "Accentuate the positive and eliminate the negative."

The lessons I learned from Jack were not only priceless, but will also stick with me forever. He treasured life, his beautiful bride of 48 years, the many friendships he had made in his long life and, so important to him, his wonderful family. If you have never heard that song, do yourself a favor and listen to it.

To sit with my new friend—a gentleman who had traveled the world, met people from all walks of life, but found just as much pleasure in sitting with me, telling stories and singing our songs as they blared throughout the house—were times that I will always cherish.

Together, we shared stories of my life, stories of his life and the true bond of our devotion to what is important... people. In him, I found a man who valued *time* well spent with family and friends more than anyone I had known since my dad.

The day my friend Jack died, I cried as though I had again lost my dad. Jack too was an Irish man. He loved golf, while my dad loved fishing, but they both had the skin worn from the days spent in the sun. Like my dad, he would drop everything to tell a story or spend *time* with anyone who wanted to share a moment, tell him a story or sing a song. I was never in his home without humming that song, smiling at the memory of him being patient with my off-key voice, and knowing that although those before him had touched my heart, he enriched my life unlike anyone else.

Irish Whiskey and Taste Buds

Being Irish myself, I could appreciate the taste of a good Irish whiskey or Irish cream (although I prefer beer); a gentleman I had the privilege of caring for preferred his Irish whiskey. It just seemed to go down smooth with a tray of cheese and crackers. Unfortunately, after some health issues, the doctor (not me blaming it on the doctor, but the real doctor) allowed only so many ounces a day. This was going to be an obstacle, as this gentleman was very independent!

I tried to make the drinks for him while adding more water than he ever did, putting it on the rocks and serving it with a positive smile. However, we Irish know our drinks, and something was not right! Thinking quickly, I blamed the dull taste on his oxygen, which was not only new to him, but could definitely "change the taste of things." This worked for a little while, until I was promptly fired from the duty of making the drinks. Knowing I needed to give him back the task of making his own drink, and also knowing I needed to abide by the doctor's orders, I began setting up what looked like a "moonshine still" in an unused bathroom of his home.

There, I would take a full bottle and evenly pour it into three other bottles with a funnel I had stashed. I then diluted all, making four bottles out of one. I would bring one bottle at a time and place it in the cupboard, where it had always been stored. When it was time to make a drink, I would offer assistance, knowing I would be told, "No thanks," and would watch as my friend made the "perfect drink, as always." I never shared this story with anyone until my friend passed away.

During a family get-together, I was asked if there was any Irish whiskey in the house. Chuckling, I said, "Of course, I will get some." Bringing a diluted bottle and a new bottle, I told the guests they were welcome to have many drinks from *this* bottle while holding up the diluted one. Or they might want to limit what they had from *this* one and held up the true Irish whiskey (undiluted bottle).

Everyone laughed and commented on how I pulled one over on our friend, but I said, "Trust me, the luck of the Irish isn't always with you. I might have been lucky to do this here, but when I see him in Heaven, I imagine he will have an O'Doul's in a frosted mug for me, and he and my dad will have a good laugh at my expense!"

Notes from the Author

As I continue to care for the many elders in my life, I have a special spot in my heart for each and every one. I carry their memory, their knowledge and the gift of friendship that each one has given to me. The comfort I gave to them is a comfort to me also, knowing that I made a difference in their lives and surely they made a difference in mine! And, although they are gone, their stories, their love and their treasures continue through me.

What a gift for all of us and all it took was *time.*

Helpful Hints

~ <u>First and foremost, get all the paperwork in order</u>. Go online to get Advanced Directives, Power of Attorney, Medical Power of Attorney and DNR (Do Not Resuscitate) forms. Then, make sure you fill them out now, before you need them. (Most of these are also available through your local state agencies.) Once completed, give a copy to your doctor.

~ <u>Get a notebook for documentation.</u> Remember, it is difficult to have someone write things about you. If the elder asks, tell him or her this is used for doctor's visits as a tool in helping to answer all of the doctor's questions.

~ <u>If a decision about a hospital bed, oxygen or something else is meeting resistance from your loved one, blame it on the doctor</u>. Unlike some people today, this generation has great confidence in doctors and usually will do what the doctor recommends.

~ <u>Always be positive</u>. Presentation is everything. If you are okay with the changes necessary, your loved one will follow your lead. Your facial expressions and body language are just as important. A smile goes a long way when trying to reassure someone.

~ Try to avoid the word "remember?" Instead, use "I recall" or "what about the time?"

~ When bathing or changing someone, always keep the area of his or her body that you are not washing covered. This allows them to retain their dignity. Also, talk to them, thereby taking their mind off of what you are doing and what they can't do for themselves.

~ Get a baby monitor. When installing a baby monitor, refer to it as an intercom or "one-way radio / walkie-talkie."

~ For the transition to adult diapers, take the panties/boxers out of the drawer and replace with Depends. Then there is no choice to make. NEVER refer to them as diapers.

~ Do not say, "Let me help you" or "I am taking care of you." This sounds needy; instead say, "Let me assist you" or "May I help you with that?"

~ Try to be conscientious of certain facts. Very important, be aware that the hardest thing for a man to lose control of is driving. For a woman, it is to lose her home or have someone come in to her home and do the things she has always done.

~ Praise the things that the elder can still accomplish. We all like to feel important and independent as possible.

~ Unlike our generation of getting second and third opinions from doctors, our parents' put their total trust in one doctor for their entire life. Therefore, when I would need my dad to take a medication or change a routine that wasn't working any longer,

I would tell him, "I talked to your doctor and the doctor recommended this," thus making Dad more accepting. It wasn't his daughter "telling" or "making" him do this; it was his doctor, so it must be okay.

~ <u>Keep a calendar handy to mark off the days as they pass and also orient your loved one to each day.</u> Circle special dates and appointments on the calendar, but not too far in advance, as this tends to be overwhelming.

~ <u>Don't allow invitations to weddings, parties, etc. to be sent directly to your loved one.</u> This causes stress and apprehension as to whether they will "remember." Instead, RSVP for them, telling the person that attempts will be made to attend but no promises made. (The decision depends on the outlook of that day.) Afford privacy by not going into detail about their condition. Simply say, "We will try." If this is not acceptable, then decline the invite.

~ <u>Never talk about personal or negative things around your loved one as though he or she is not there.</u> Instead, look into his or her eyes, and you will see he or she is "still in there," sometimes just unable to respond. Give the respect and privacy he or she deserves. If you need to discuss something sensitive with the doctor, sibling, etc., excuse yourself, saying you will be right back and then address it in another room. Make it short since this causes paranoia as to why he or she can't know what is being discussed.

~ Keep in mind our parents have lost many things at this point. This includes spouse, home, driving privilege, job, friends, neighborhood, etc. Don't take away their ability to control what they still can. Simply present only two choices of clothing to wear; specify two times to leave for an outing (nine o'clock or ten o'clock); two different items for dinner (fried chicken with potatoes or rice); two times for bedtime and so on. Imagine, if everything were decided for you, what would be the point of working your mind? Actually, give simple or mini tasks to stimulate their mind and then the proper *time* to accomplish them, making sure it is in Alzheimer's *time,* not clock *time.*

~ Occasionally, out-of-town friends or family will ride into town, like the cavalry, ready to make changes and "fix" everything before they ride out. Remember, they are struggling too. Their job of helping is limited because of the distance; they mean well but can only do so much. Accept their ideas, listen to what they say and implement anything helpful. Or change nothing—it ultimately is your daily routine and responsibility, and they know you are doing your best.

~ Always, and I repeat always, give your loved one *time* to respond. When you ask a question or are holding a conversation that warrants a response, make sure you wait to get a response. I have found we are sometimes impatient with the silence of no response. When, in reality, our parent is just taking *time* to process what you have said or asked and then thinking about the answer and how to get that thought process into speech. This takes *time,* especially when you are searching through 90 years of memories to get that answer... just be patient.

~ <u>If it is *time* for your friend or family member to die, give him or her permission</u>. It is important for everyone to know that the ones you leave behind are going to be okay.

~ <u>After they are gone, continue their legacy with all the wonderful stories they left you.</u> I have now come to know the pain of losing my parents and can say to you, after you lose a parent, you will never be the same, but you will be okay. Different, but okay.

~ <u>Most important, take one day at a *time*</u>! And, if today doesn't go well, there is always tomorrow. Enjoy the happy times and learn by the struggles!

A Few Closing Thoughts

In caring for the many elderly people I have an continue to in my life, there has been one thing they all have in common: their physical appearance. When you first see an elderly person, you are aware of the wrinkled skin from years of struggles and accomplishments. The eyes are filled with wisdom and knowledge. One's physical body, possibly not cooperating as well, now needs the assistance from a walker or wheelchair. Hands have aged from the years of hard work or the midday sun from fishing, as my dad's had been.

I too see these things, but I also see something different. Their eyes are filled with the memories of the little-girl giggles or the little-boy mischief. And all are filled with a lifetime of *treasures*. In talking and spending *time* with my lovely aged friends, I have come to know that we miss out when we don't take the *time* to ask questions. To tell one of our stories that will spark a memory of their youth and promote one of their stories, which in turn brings such wonder to them from a memory that hadn't been told for a "very long *time*." I have found when sharing just a portion of a situation that I recall, I can see the wheels turning in their head… through their eyes. It might take a while to get the memory out, to find the proper words to express their treasured memory, but when it does come out, it is with utter joy and excitement that, again, they have recalled this "Wonderful Moment in *Time.*"

The word *remember* is not often used by me when addressing my elderly friends. It seems when they hear that word, there is an automatic pressure put on them "to remember." Instead, I use the word *recall* or use a sentence, such as, "I had a dog named Patches when I was a little girl; did you ever have a dog?" And then, most important, I give them the *time* to think about it and tell me their answer.

So often when someone, especially an elderly person, is asked a question, we tend to answer for him or her. We don't have to answer for them; we just need to wait and pause, giving him or her the *time* to gather his or her thoughts to then put them into words.

Let's not forget that we are talking to people just like us— the same people who used to disobey their parents, pull pranks on their siblings or friends, tried to hide a bad grade from school, experienced young love, or got nervous for their first kiss or their honeymoon night. People who are no different from you or me, just older, wiser and needing assistance. I try to remember, while I can, that I too will be older, hopefully wiser, and possibly needing assistance. If I do need assistance, I would like to know that someone will take the *time* to hear my stories, ask about my friends and family and know that in these eyes they carry a lifetime of wonderful stories from someone who has seen a lot, lived a lot and gathered information from those who did the same, long before I was ever born.

I have referenced the word *time* approximately 235 places in my book. Initially, I thought this should be changed. In hindsight, I decided to make the word italicized to bring attention to it. Often, I am drawn to remind people, who are in the situation as I was with my dad and now am with my profession, that *time* can be your best friend when your vacation is going by slowly and every moment is relaxing. Or *time* can be your worst enemy when you are afflicted with the disability of Alzheimer's or being dependent on your family. Embrace the *time* either way and know just as that vacation will end, so will your parents' needs.... don't rush either.

During my story, I never used a name or picture of my dad, as I don't want these thoughts to only be about my parent. It can be anyone's loved one with Alzheimer's or the aging process as a whole. The ideas and theories are the same, and we all need encouragement throughout this journey.

Hopefully, you will find something in these words—an idea you might want to try, a thought that never occurred to you or maybe just some words of comfort from someone who's been where you are and can understand where you are going. Most important, remember to always enjoy and treasure the *time* you spend with the ones you love.

About the Author

After putting her career on hold to take care of her dad during a time when he needed additional care, Trisha Waskey learned firsthand the struggle of dementia and Alzheimer's. After her father's passing in December 2002, she realized that she needed to do something with her knowledge. She went to the local community college and earned her CNA (Certified Nursing Assistant), GNA (Geriatric Nursing Assistant) and Medication Technician licenses. This allowed her to continue her work in elder care. Since 2002, she has actively worked in assisted-living facilities, provided in-home health care and taught seminars on working with the elderly. Her work continues today.